OXFORD SPECIALTY TRAINING

Self-Assessment for the MC

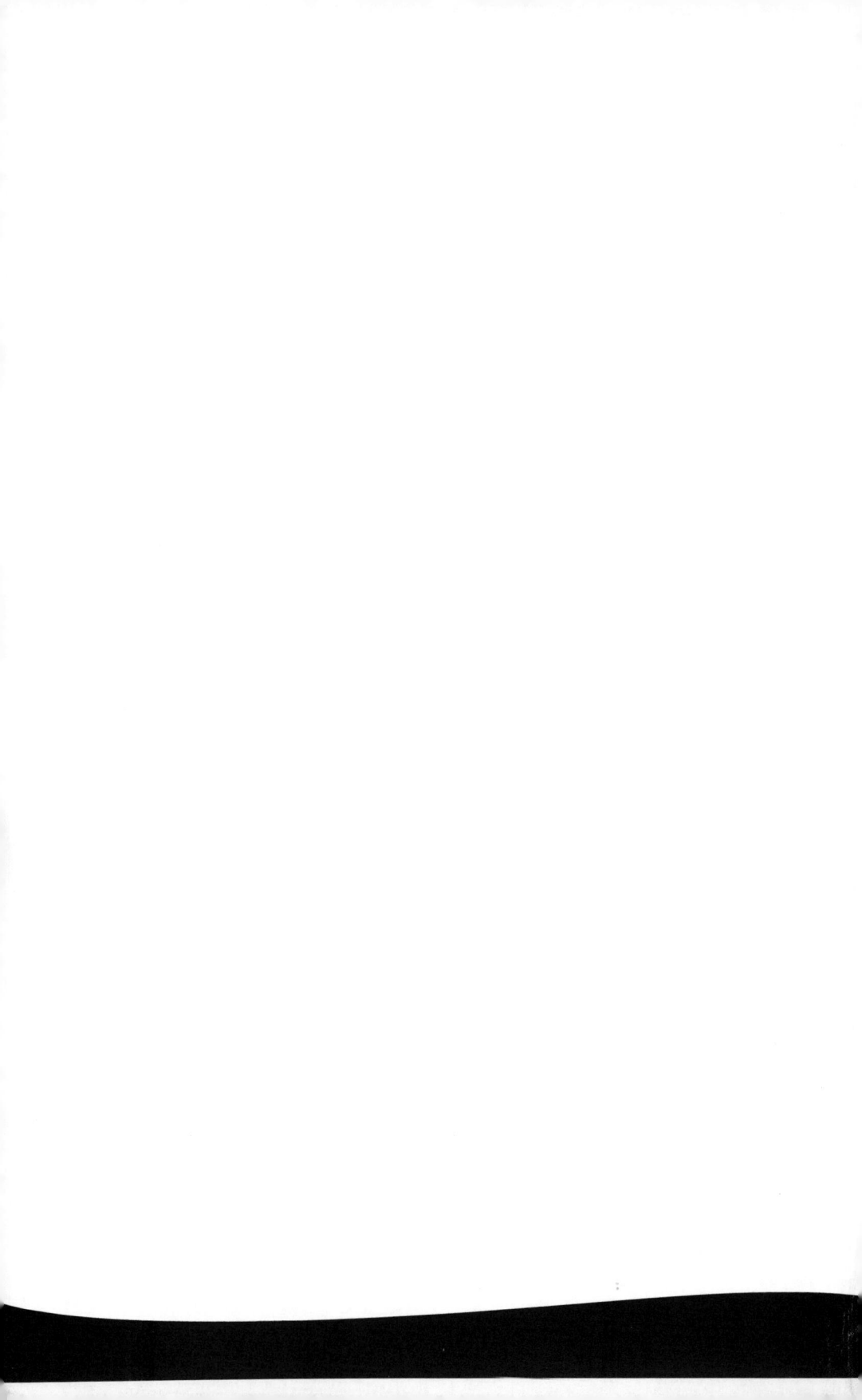

OXFORD SPECIALTY TRAINING

Self-Assessment for the MCEM Part C

Dr Rebecca Thorpe
Consultant in Emergency Medicine, University Hospitals Bristol NHS Foundation Trust, Bristol

Dr Simon Chapman
Consultant in Emergency Medicine, Jersey General Hospital, Jersey

Dr Jules Blackham
Consultant in Emergency Medicine, North Bristol Trust, Bristol

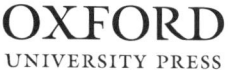

OXFORD
UNIVERSITY PRESS

Great Clarendon Street, Oxford, OX2 6DP,
United Kingdom

Oxford University Press is a department of the University of Oxford.
It furthers the University's objective of excellence in research, scholarship,
and education by publishing worldwide. Oxford is a registered trade mark of
Oxford University Press in the UK and in certain other countries

© Oxford University Press 2014

The moral rights of the authors have been asserted

First Edition published in 2014

All rights reserved. No part of this publication may be reproduced, stored in
a retrieval system, or transmitted, in any form or by any means, without the
prior permission in writing of Oxford University Press, or as expressly permitted
by law, by licence or under terms agreed with the appropriate reprographics
rights organization. Enquiries concerning reproduction outside the scope of the
above should be sent to the Rights Department, Oxford University Press, at the
address above

You must not circulate this work in any other form
and you must impose this same condition on any acquirer

Published in the United States of America by Oxford University Press
198 Madison Avenue, New York, NY 10016, United States of America

British Library Cataloguing in Publication Data
Data available

Library of Congress Control Number: 2014942349

ISBN 978–0–19–871758–4

Oxford University Press makes no representation, express or implied, that the
drug dosages in this book are correct. Readers must therefore always check
the product information and clinical procedures with the most up-to-date
published product information and data sheets provided by the manufacturers
and the most recent codes of conduct and safety regulations. The authors and
the publishers do not accept responsibility or legal liability for any errors in the
text or for the misuse or misapplication of material in this work. Except where
otherwise stated, drug dosages and recommendations are for the non-pregnant
adult who is not breast-feeding

Links to third party websites are provided by Oxford in good faith and
for information only. Oxford disclaims any responsibility for the materials
contained in any third party website referenced in this work.

Foreword

The MCEM C examination is a 'rite of passage'. Success demonstrates that the candidate has the requisite knowledge, skills, and understanding of the practice of emergency medicine to progress confidently into higher specialist training. The examination is both comprehensive and rigorous; in consequence all successful candidates should be rightly proud of their achievement.

Such success can only be achieved by a combination of experience and education; neither alone can properly prepare the candidate for the challenge of the MCEM examination. The famous Canadian physician Sir William Osler made many astute observations regarding the practice of medicine, none more so than 'He who studies medicine without books sails an uncharted sea'.

This book, written by three practicing EM consultants with first hand knowledge of the experience of the MCEM examination will provide the necessary chart to plan your revision and ensure proper coverage of the curriculum.

This book does not simply describe the requisite knowledge and skills but includes a full description of the approach to each OSCE, including examples of how the marks are awarded and the relevant emphasis of each station. As such the text gives a real insight into the methodology of each major question type and enables the candidate to fully appreciate what is expected of them and hence allows the reader to optimize their approach to each OSCE.

In an OSCE examination it is seldom the case that errors are the cause of failure. It is almost always omissions that prevent the candidate from gaining sufficient marks to pass. The real strength of this book is that it focuses on ensuring such omissions are avoided. As such it allows the candidate to make best use of their knowledge and skills, rather than adding to the burden of 'fact retention'.

The 100 practice examination questions cover the eight main categories of OSCE seen in the MCEM. Whilst no text book can guarantee examination success it is inconceivable that armed with the knowledge derived from this book, any candidate would not be better prepared.

Dr. Clifford J. Mann FCEM FRCP
President of the College of Emergency Medicine

Contents

Questions by Subject ix
Abbreviations xiii

Section 1 **Introduction** *1*

Section 2 **Questions** *11*

Index 227

Questions by Subject

Resuscitation Questions

Question 2	Neonatal resuscitation
Question 34	Airway skills
Question 35	Obstetric emergency
Question 38	Shortness of breath 2
Question 40	Paediatric trauma
Question 41	Choking
Question 52	Airway management
Question 59	Basic Life Support
Question 69	Hypothermia
Question 70	Infant resuscitation
Question 72	Burns
Question 73	Anaphylaxis
Question 76	Seizure 3
Question 79	Poisoning
Question 81	Sepsis
Question 87	Asystole
Question 97	Seizure 4

Examination Questions

Question 3	Cardiovascular examination
Question 19	Shoulder examination
Question 23	Respiratory system examination
Question 27	Knee examination
Question 33	Neck injury 1
Question 37	Eye examination
Question 46	Cranial nerve examination
Question 47	Peripheral nervous system
Question 49	Wrist examination
Question 51	Elbow injury
Question 54	Neck injury 2
Question 57	Ankle injury
Question 66	Hand examination
Question 67	Abdominal examination
Question 75	Pelvic examination

Practicals and Procedures

Question 4	Catheterization
Question 6	Chest aspiration
Question 8	Paronychia
Question 10	Forearm plaster
Question 14	ECG
Question 17	Knee joint aspiration
Question 21	Suturing

Questions by Subject

Question 32	Femoral line
Question 34	Airway skills
Question 48	Ankle plaster
Question 51	Elbow injury
Question 58	Ultrasound
Question 60	Chest drain
Question 63	Arterial line
Question 68	Lumbar puncture
Question 86	Central line
Question 88	Facial wound
Question 95	Intraosseus line
Question 96	Wound closure
Question 100	Foreign body removal

Teaching Questions

Question 18	Auroscopy
Question 39	Ophthalmoscopy
Question 82	ECG
Question 83	Deep vein thrombosis
Question 91	Blood gas analysis

History-taking Questions

Question 1	Emergency gynaecology
Question 7	Returning traveller
Question 11	Sickle cell disease
Question 13	Chest pain 1
Question 16	Psychiatry
Question 20	Overdose
Question 22	Shortness of breath 1
Question 24	Child protection
Question 28	Chest pain 2
Question 29	Headache
Question 30	Ear pain
Question 31	Diarrhoea and vomiting
Question 36	Risk assessment in overdose
Question 43	Limping child
Question 45	Dysuria
Question 55	Seizure 1
Question 57	Ankle injury
Question 65	Abdominal pain 2
Question 71	Seizure 2
Question 80	Mental state examination
Question 90	Needlestick injury
Question 92	Jaundice
Question 94	Haematemesis
Question 99	Syncope

Breaking Bad News Questions

Question 9	Breaking bad news 1
Question 25	Breaking bad news 2
Question 44	Breaking bad news 3
Question 61	Organ donation
Question 84	Breaking bad news 4

Explanatory Questions

Question 5	Pulled elbow
Question 11	Sickle cell
Question 12	Error
Question 24	Child protection
Question 26	Asthma
Question 29	Headache
Question 30	Ear pain
Question 42	Capacity
Question 43	Limping child
Question 49	Wrist injury
Question 50	Handover
Question 53	Sedation
Question 54	Neck injury 2
Question 56	Regional anaesthesia
Question 57	Ankle injury
Question 61	Organ donation
Question 62	Inhaler technique
Question 64	Abdominal pain 1
Question 74	Antibiotic requesting
Question 75	Pelvic examination
Question 77	Vaginal bleeding
Question 78	Febrile convulsion
Question 89	Dehydration
Question 90	Needlestick injury
Question 93	Driving advice
Question 98	Septic screen
Question 99	Syncope

Referral Questions

Question 15	Neurosurgical referral
Question 85	Aortic aneurysm

Abbreviations

'4 Hs'	hypothermia, hypoxia, hypotension, hypo/hyperkalaemia
'4 Ts'	tamponade (cardiac), tension pneumothorax, toxic, thromboembolic
AAA	abdominal aortic aneurysm
ABC	airway, breathing, and circulation
ACJ	acromioclavicular joint
BE	base excess
BHCG	beta human chorionic gonadotrophin (urine and blood levels used in pregnancy testing)
BP	blood pressure
bpm	beats per minute
BVM	bag valve mask
CCTV	closed circuit television
CEM	College of Emergency Medicine
CPN	Community Psychiatric Nurse
CPR	cardiopulmonary resuscitation
CRT	capillary refill time
CSF	cerebrospinal fluid
CT	computerized topography
CXR	chest X-ray
DC	direct current
DVLA	Driver and Vehicle Licensing Agency
DVT	deep vein thrombosis
ECG	electrocardiogram
ED	Emergency Department
EM	emergency medicine
ENT	ears, nose, throat
EPO	erythropoeitin
ERCP	endoscopic retrograde cholangiopancreatography
$ETCO_2$	end tidal carbon dioxide
ETT	endotracheal tube
F2	Foundation Year 2 doctor
FAST	focused assessment with sonography for trauma
GA	general anaesthesia
GCS	Glasgow Coma Scale
GI	gastrointestinal
GP	General Practitioner
GTN	glyceryl trinitrate
GUM	genito-urinary medicine
HR	heart rate

Abbreviations

IM	intramuscular
IO	intraosseus
ITU	Intensive Therapy Unit
IV	intravenous
IVF	in-vitro fertilization
JVP	jugular venous pressure
LMA	laryngeal mask airway
LP	lumbar puncture
MAP	morning after pill
MCPJ	metacarpal-phalangeal joint
MC&S	microscopy, culture, and sensitivity
MRI	magnetic resonance imaging
MTPJ	metatarsal-phalangeal joint
NAI	non-accidental injury
NIBP	non-invasive blood pressure
NICE	National Institute for Health and Care Excellence
NOF	neck of femur
NP	nasopharyngeal
NSAID	non-steroidal anti-inflammatory drug
OETT	oral endotracheal tube
OP	oropharyngeal
pCO_2	partial pressure of carbon dioxide
PE	pulmonary embolism
PEA	pulseless electrical activity
PICU	paediatric intensive care unit
PIP	proximal interphalangeal
pO_2	partial pressure of oxygen
resus	resuscitation room of Emergency Department
RR	respiratory rate
RSI	rapid sequence induction (of anaesthesia)
SaO_2	oxygen saturations
SBAR	situation, background, assessment, recommendation
SHO	Senior House Officer
SOB	shortness of breath
STI	sexually transmitted infection
U&E	urea and electrolytes
USS	ultrasound scan
VBG	venous blood gas
VF	ventricular fibrillation
VT	ventricular tachycardia
WBC	white blood cells

Section 1 **Introduction**

What is the purpose of this book?

This book has been written by Consultants in Emergency Medicine (EM) as an aid to doctors studying for the Membership of the College of Emergency Medicine (MCEM) Part C: Objective Structured Clinical Examination (OSCE) Examination. It provides an invaluable guide and companion to this section of the MCEM examination. One hundred example OSCEs are provided for prospective candidates to review. Each question consists of detailed information that allows candidates to appreciate the format and requirements of each OSCE. The 2010 College of Emergency Medicine (CEM) curriculum has been used to ensure that each OSCE has been mapped against specific competencies. Candidate, examiner, and patient actor information is provided, as well as equipment lists allowing readers to recreate OSCE stations for practice if they so wish. MCEM-style[1] marking sheets ensure that readers have a good understanding of the standard required by the CEM.

Approach to the MCEM Part C exam

As with all parts of the examination process it is vital that candidates familiarize themselves with the most recent CEM examination guidelines, available on the College website prior to each exam diet.
The College states that:

> The Membership Examination assesses the knowledge, skills and behaviours necessary for the clinical practice of Emergency Medicine in the UK and Ireland, at the level of the senior decision maker. This is defined currently as the equivalent of the ST4 or specialty doctor. The standard is at a level suitable to supervise foundation and core trainees and to provide senior clinical decision making when there is no consultant presence in the department.
>
> In particular Part C assesses the knowledge and clinical competences required for the evaluation and immediate management of common clinical conditions seen in the Emergency department. The full breadth of the major and acute presentations listed in the curriculum can be tested. Competence in children's emergencies is expected at a level delivered in a general Emergency Department and focuses mainly on the seriously ill and injured child, or the management of common childhood emergencies.

The College has provided some additional information in relation to the Part C exam and this has been included where relevant in the text boxes.

MCEM Part C is the final part of the MCEM examination and provides the opportunity for candidates to demonstrate their clinical acumen in simulated clinical encounters. It consists of 18 OSCE stations over the course of 2.5 hours. There will normally be two rest stations.

The College uses these simulated clinical encounters to ensure that candidates have achieved a sufficient level of clinical knowledge to enter higher specialist training. However, knowledge in itself does not form the fundamental requirements of success in the OSCE format and various performance domains are evaluated. Key performance domains that are assessed include:

- knowledge
- clinical decision-making skills
- psycho-motor ability
- attitude

---

[1] Please note that the authors are not MCEM examiners.

- interpersonal skills (including communication and conflict resolution)
- professional behaviour

Candidates are required to pass 14 of the 18 stations to pass the whole examination.

Format of the MCEM Part C exam

Preparation
The OSCE is best considered as an act of 7 minutes' duration. It takes place in a specific setting, and requires certain dialogue and specific actions. To succeed, it is best to consider it in terms of an entrance, middle, and exit.

Setting
The examination will usually take place in a large single room that will be set up with a series of partitioned makeshift cubicles. Candidates line up outside the examination room, and when they are allowed to enter each will be given a specific cubicle to wait outside of.

Dress code
The examination assesses your clinical practice. You will be more at ease if you are dressed in your usual clinical attire—cleaned and ironed though! See Box 1.1.

Box 1.1 CEM advice—*What can I wear to an OSCE?*

Smart attire is expected for the exam but the College is happy for you to wear scrubs in the OSCE if you feel more comfortable. You will not be admitted to the exam, however, if you arrive wearing scrubs, and will not be able to go outside for a cigarette while wearing scrubs.

Instructions
On the wall of the cubicle there will be a typed sheet containing the key details of the station and task that is required. It will also broadly indicate which competencies are being tested, depicted by a pie chart.

One minute is provided to allow the candidate to prepare prior to commencing each station. A bell will then ring to indicate the start of the examination. See Boxes Box 1.2 and 1.3.

Box 1.2 CEM advice—*What if I am not clear about the task in a station?*

Each station will have clear instructions outside, not only setting the clinical scenario but also a separate line for 'task'. In addition there will be a pie chart of the breakdown of skills that is being examined, i.e. clinical examination, communication skills, diagnostic reasoning.

An example of the type of instructions provided is shown in Box 1.3.

Format of the MCEM Part C exam

Box 1.3 Example of instructions provided for candidate

Instructions for the candidate for suturing station
A 20-year-old builder (Mr Jones) has sustained a laceration to his right upper arm on a piece of sheet metal while at work. The wound is not dirty and suitable for primary closure. There is no neurovascular deficit or foreign body.

Task
Briefly confirm the history with the patient and close the wound using the equipment supplied. You should advise the patient on the care of his wound and removal of sutures.

Examiner's role
Observation and time keeping.

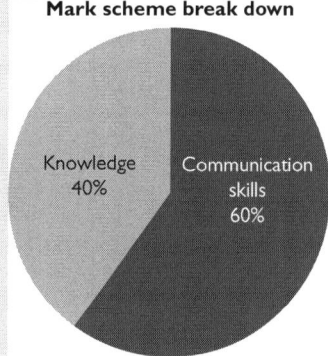

There is also a copy of the candidate instructions inside the station and the examiner will reiterate as you go in the station what the task is. If you are in any doubt, clarify before you start.

Preparation

At the start of each OSCE, you will be allowed 1 minute before entering the station, during which you must:

- read thoroughly and completely the information provided
- ask yourself which competency is being tested
- focus on doing your best on this station

A bell will ring after 1 minute.

Entrance

At the bell an examiner should invite you into the cubicle. If they don't, then knock and enter. In the cubicle you will find two examiners: one will lead the station and the other will observe/carry out the marking. There may also be a patient/actor and whatever pertinent equipment is required for the station.

First impressions count

The examiners will assess a significant number of candidates during the day. Candidates who enter looking nervous or unsure will undoubtedly be under more scrutiny during the station than those who enter in a confident and self-assured manner. It is therefore worth spending some time rehearsing an opening introductory dialogue. This should become your standard opening introduction that you use for most stations. A well-delivered introduction conveys self-assurance and allows you to control the start of the OSCE, settles nerves, as well as providing time for you to gather your thoughts before commencing the specific competency. The introduction can be used to cover generic points of patient comfort, analgesia, chaperones, and hand washing—ensuring that easy marks are scored in a timely and consistent fashion (see Box 1.4).

> **Box 1.4** CEM advice—*Should I introduce myself as I go in to a station?*
>
> *This can be confusing, as the scenario may suggest that you have already examined the patient, or taken a history, and so it does not seem natural to introduce or recap. However, for the sake of the integrity of the station, and bearing in mind the need to demonstrate professional skills, we would recommend that you do introduce yourself, and indeed recap on what you have been told in the scenario before commencing the next bit of the patient management. Hence in a station providing advice on a given diagnosis, you would always revisit the diagnosis to check what the patient has been told. The station may be constructed so that you have taken over from a Senior House Officer (SHO), so it is natural to introduce and recap, but occasionally you have to suspend your disbelief and just act as if you have just met the patient!*

Perform the competency that you have been directed to perform. It is very easy to lose sight of this when confronted with a patient actor. It is imperative to utilize the 1 minute reading time to focus on the specific objective that you are required to perform. You should adopt a 'driving test' mentality. You are performing each competency in order to demonstrate your abilities, rather than managing a real clinical case. Therefore you must ensure that the examiners are fully aware of what you are doing and why you are doing it (see Box 1.5).

> **Box 1.5** CEM advice—*Should I talk aloud in an OSCE?*
>
> *If you are in an examination station, and the station does not include a section at the end for you to give the examiner your findings, then you should say out loud what you are doing as you do it. This helps the examiner to be clear that you are performing each task. The examiner can only give you a mark for doing something if s/he sees and understands clearly that you are doing it.*

In each station, the examiner(s) will use a predefined competency check list on which to score the candidate, including a 'global score' component (see Box 1.6). Be mindful of this in your approach to the OSCE station, and concentrate on maintaining exemplary behaviour at all times.

> **Box 1.6** CEM advice—*What is the global score?*
>
> *The global score is a mark out of 5 given by the examiner (and the role player where relevant) that gives a mark for your 'professionalism'. Reading the matrix is useful as you will see that you get marks for the unspoken communications, the way you ask questions, aspects of team leadership, etc. This global score is added to the marks for the task itself, and so you can score a proportion of your marks easily if you know what professional behaviours examiners are looking for. The matrix is provided in Table 1.1.*

Timing

Single stations are 7 minutes long from bell to bell. It is best to practice OSCEs in real time in order to get a good feel for the pace of each particular competency. On some occasions, examiners will indicate that you should stop and summarize your findings, but this should not be counted on. It is therefore advantageous to be able to complete examinations within 6 minutes to allow time to present findings, summarize management plans, and answer any specific questions that the examiners or patient actors may have.

Exit

When the end of bell goes thank everyone in the cubicle and walk out to the next station. However badly you think the last station went, put this to one side to start the next station afresh.

When you arrive at the next station there will be a typed A4 sheet containing the details of the scenario and the specific task that you are required to perform. You have 1 minute. You absolutely must:

- read thoroughly and completely the information provided
- ask yourself which competency is being tested
- focus on doing your best on this station—put the previous station behind you—focus on what is being assessed on the current station. See Box 1.7.

Box 1.7 CEM advice—*What if I finish a station early?*

There are some stations where it is common to finish before the bell. Do not be alarmed. In a scenario station, the examiner will say, 'You have completed the scenario'. Alternatively, in the history taking or communication stations the examiner may ask you if you have finished. We would recommend that you stay in the station until the bell, since you may remember something you would have wanted to say and can mention it and still get marks. Remember, it is your time.

Out of 18 stations each candidate is required to pass 14.

The most important point to keep in mind is that each station is marked individually—compartmentalize, move on, reset, and focus (see Boxes Box 1.8 and 1.9).

Box 1.8 CEM advice—*Do I have to pass each question or station?*

The OSCE is marked so that you can fail a number of stations (the equivalent of four, provided they are not both of the double stations) and each station is pass/fail individually.

Box 1.9 *Are there any critical questions, stations, or individual parts of questions or stations that mean I will fail the exam?*

Within the MCEM there are no 'sudden death' or critical response questions or actions. This means that there is no one thing that you can do in the OSCE that will result in an automatic fail.

What to expect

The College designs OSCEs to cover key competencies:

- Taking a history
- Clinical examination of a system
- Clinical examination of a joint
- Demonstration of a clinical (practical) skill
- Team leadership
- Resuscitation skills
- Teaching skills
- Difficult communication interaction

Actors

The OSCEs are scripted to follow a certain path. Patient actors are routinely used and patients with stable clinical signs are used in clinical examination stations. It must be appreciated that patient actors may mimic clinical signs to varying degrees of accuracy. Similarly, candidates should appreciate the limitations of equipment provided and the varying degree in which disbelief may need to be suspended. Remember that you are demonstrating to the examiners that you have the appropriate clinical ability; do not get distracted by limitations of equipment, the realism of manikins, or quality of images. See Boxes 1.10 and 1.11.

> **Box 1.10** CEM advice—*What do I do in a team resus scenario?*
>
> *The resus stations will be set up either as a small junior team where you will be clearly required to do some of the procedures yourself (i.e. all-nurse team) or as a team whereby there are skills in the team members and your leadership skills are being tested. Remember to check the pie chart to see which it is, and if leadership is being tested, keep your hands off the patient! An important tip when you feel desperately short of hands is to consider if you are using the given helpers properly. Have you released the neck immobilizer for example?*

> **Box 1.11** *If it is a teaching station, do I have to do the whole four-step approach as in ATLS?*
>
> *The stations are not really long enough for this. The College is not wishing to see any particular method of teaching, other than the ability to explain simply and carefully the skill involved and to check the student has taken in the instruction. Therefore talking as you demonstrate a skill and then allowing the student to practise is acceptable.*

OSCE do's

- Appearance
  - Clothing—wear what you would at work—smart and ironed
  - Be quietly confident and appear calm at all times
  - Maintain dignified humility
- Read all the information—you have been given it for a reason
- Reread all the information—make sure that you know the task that you are required to achieve

- Listen—very carefully to the examiners and patient actors
- Observe—be aware of non-verbal clues—examiners/patient actors may inadvertently give you pointers by their behaviour
- Be polite to everybody prior to and during the exam; they may well be a patient actor!
- Be attentive and listen to the patient actor—they have been given a script for a reason
- Make sure that you ask the patient actor if they have any questions
- First impressions count—always start positively with a good friendly introduction
- Be structured in your assessment and summaries—keep information relevant
- Think before you speak
- Be safe and conventional in your management plans—remember, this is what you do as an Emergency physician; have a safe recognizable approach to your OSCE and make sure that the examiners are given the opportunity to observe and hear this
- Aim to finish with enough time to provide a summary of findings and an outline of ongoing management plans, as well as giving the opportunity to answer questions—these all count as scoring opportunities
- When you finish a station—put it to one side and concentrate on the next station—you only have 1 minute to evaluate the next OSCE task.

OSCE don'ts

- Be rude, loud, or arrogant—be a nice, confident senior doctor
- Be dismissive of the exam—treat the exam with respect and suspend disbelief—the stations/manikins/images will not be 'perfect'
- Argue—be firm with patient actors when you need to be—but don't be rude or dismissive. Remember, the examiner is always right. If they give you direction—listen and follow it
- Hurt the patient
- Swear
- Panic or freeze. If in doubt then verbally recap the situation so far—the examiners will think that you have a structured approach, the patient actor will think that you have been listening, and you will give yourself time to think
- Worry about other candidates' performances. The examiners can subtlety change OSCE details; AF becomes SVT, etc.—so ignore what you may overhear or what other candidates may say
- Worry if you forget specific terminology or eponymous names—explain what you mean
- Don't get too worried—remember, this is what you do day by day as an Emergency physician

Matrix for awarding the global score

The following text and the Global Scoring Matrix are reproduced with the kind permission of the College of Emergency Medicine.

This matrix sets out indicative behaviour in generic domains of professional behaviour (Table 1.1). It should be used by the examiners and the role player where appropriate to determine the global score. Not every domain will be applicable to every skill station. Please use the matrix to identify the global score. As a rough rule:

5 = mostly exemplary
4 = mix of exemplary and acceptable
3 = mostly acceptable
2 = mix of acceptable and unacceptable
1 = mostly unacceptable

Table 1.1 Global scoring matrix

	Examples of unacceptable behaviour	Examples of acceptable behaviour	Examples of exemplary behaviour
Communication	No introduction, and no information about what the station is about	Attempts to introduce themselves and to inform what about to do	Introduces and informs what the task is about
	Closed questions	Some open questions	Open and closed questions used appropriately
	Not listening to the answer	Invites questions	Good use of silence
	Gives the answer themselves	Occasionally interrupts inappropriately	Invites questions from patient and answers well in plain English
	Doesn't' warn patient of actions	Attempts to explain what is doing	Keeps patient involved and informed constantly
	Uses jargon without explanation	Uses jargon but then explains	
Rapport and empathy	No attempt to establish rapport	Adequate rapport	Excellent rapport
	No response to body language or patient distress	Responds to distress but obviously uncomfortable, no eye contact	Empathic, good eye contact
		Didn't offend but not always mindful of patient privacy or comfort	Appropriate body language
	Hurts or embarrasses patient		Ensures patient comfort
Professional competence	Appears novice	Logical structure but halting and stilted	Logical sequence
	No structure to task		Looks polished
	Steps in wrong order	Has to pause to think	Confident
	Appears over/underconfident	Appears under confident	Appears calm and professional
	Becomes uncomfortable or irritated	Clearly anxious but able to control	
Pacing	Does not complete task	Appears hurried but completes task	Completes task within time and looks comfortable
Equal opportunities/ discrimination	Appears biased—exhibits racism, sexism, or ageism	No apparent prejudice	Open, non-judgemental Actively accepting of patient's cultural or behavioural differences
	Stereotypes patients in questions and answers		
	Rude or patronizing		
Team skills	No involvement of helper	Some involvement with team/helper but works autonomously	Involves team/helper, maintains cohesive working environment
	Doesn't listen to examiners or team		
		No interaction with examiner	Interacts well with examiner, accepting given cues

Standard equipment for resuscitation scenarios

Adult equipment

Adult manikin
Cardiac monitor
Defibrillator with pads
Bag valve mask
Oro-pharyngeal airway adjuncts
Naso-pharyngeal airway adjuncts
Endotracheal tubes in selection of sizes
Stylet
Bougie
Stethoscope
Tube ties or tape
Suction catheters in selection of sizes
Wall-mounted suction
Laryngoscopes in selection of sizes
Laryngeal mask airways in selection of sizes
Resuscitation drugs
Cannulae for intravenous access
Intraosseus access
Intravenous fluids including simulated blood products
Selection of needles and syringes
Cervical collars in selection of sizes
Blankets (can also be used as wedge for pregnant patients)
Pelvic binder
Personal protective equipment (gloves, apron, mask, visor)
Thermometer
Burns dressings
Scalpels

Paediatric equipment

Child or infant manikin
Infant and child hats
Cardiac monitor
Defibrillator with pads
Bag valve mask
Oro-pharyngeal airway adjuncts
Naso-pharyngeal airway adjuncts
Endotracheal tubes in selection of sizes
Stylet
Bougie
Stethoscope
Tube ties or tape
Suction catheters in selection of sizes
Wall-mounted suction
Laryngoscopes in selection of sizes

Laryngeal mask airways in selection of sizes
Resuscitation drugs
Cannulae for intravenous access
Intraosseus access
Intravenous fluids including simulated blood products
Selection of needles and syringes
Cervical collars in selection of sizes
Blankets (can also be used as wedge for pregnant patients)
Pelvic binder
Personal protective equipment (gloves, apron, mask, visor)
Thermometer
Burns dressings
Scalpels

Section 2 **Questions**

Question 1 Emergency gynaecology

Instructions for candidate
An 18-year-old university student has attended the Emergency Department (ED) to request emergency contraception. It is a Sunday evening and none of the local pharmacies are open. Please take a history and explain to the patient what you advise her to do.

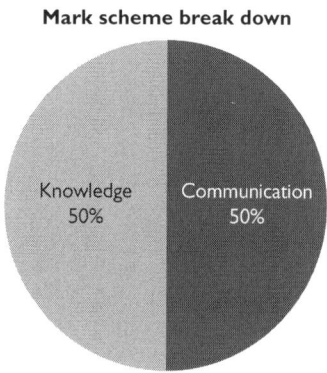

Mark scheme break down

Knowledge 50%
Communication 50%

Instructions for actor
You are an 18-year-old university student who has come to the ED to get the morning after pill (MAP). It is Sunday evening. You had unprotected sex on Saturday night at a party. You had been drinking beer and spirits all evening and don't know the boy who you had sex with. You met him at the party and know nothing about him, not even his name. You haven't come in earlier because you were 'too hung-over' during the day. You have had a few similar experiences at parties since starting university and have never used contraception. Your last period was 2 weeks ago. You have never had tests for sexually transmitted diseases. You aren't worried about catching HIV and other infections. You regularly get so drunk that you can't remember what has happened. You just want to have the pill and go home. You are willing to accept advice from the doctor and agree with what they recommend.

Instructions for examiner
Observation only.

Equipment required
None

Curriculum mapping
Sections of the CEM (2010) curriculum relevant to this question include the following.

Common competencies

CC1 History taking
CC2 Clinical examination

Self-Assessment for the MCEM Part C

CC3 Therapeutics and safe prescribing
CC4 Time management and decision-making
CC5 Decision-making and clinical reasoning
CC6 Patient as the central focus of care
CC10 Infection control
CC12 Relationship with patients and communication
CC16 Health promotion and public health
CC17 Ethics and confidentiality

Guidelines available

http://www.fpa.org.uk/helpandadvice/contraception/emergencycontraception

Mark scheme

Introduces self	1
Uses an open question to start	1
Asks exact circumstances	1
Asks if consensual sex (in order to check that this was not a sexual assault)	1
Asks if protection used	1
Confirms date of last menstrual period	1
Asks if usually sexually active	1
Asks if usually uses contraception	1
Asks about sexually transmitted infections (STIs)/testing	1
Asks about intravenous (IV) drug use	1
Discusses blood-borne viruses including hepatitis B and C, and HIV	1
Explains potential risk of viruses	1
Explains risks of sexually transmitted diseases, e.g. infertility	1
Requests urine pregnancy test	1
Explains why urine test needed	1
Explains can have MAP if pregnancy test negative	1
Advises about alcohol use by 'CAGE' or 'Paddington' test	1
(For full details of both CAGE and Paddington screening tests, go to http://www.alcohollearningcentre.org.uk/)	
Advises genito-urinary medicine (GUM) clinic review	1
Discusses contraception types available:	
• Intrauterine device	1
• Pill	1
Plans to discuss HIV/hepatitis risk with local virology expert	1
Asks if any questions	1
Global score from examiner	5
Global score from actor	5
Total	**32**

Question 2 Neonatal resuscitation

Instructions for candidate

You are the ED registrar on nights in a busy district general hospital. The delivery suite is at the other end of the hospital. Someone has just given birth in the ED car park. The sister in charge gets the woman into a bed in the resuscitation room of the ED (resus), takes the baby, and cuts the umbilical cord. She hands you the baby and attends to the mother. Please demonstrate how you would assess the newborn baby, and treat any problems that you discover. You have one experienced ED nurse with you. The baby can be assumed to weigh 3.5 kg.

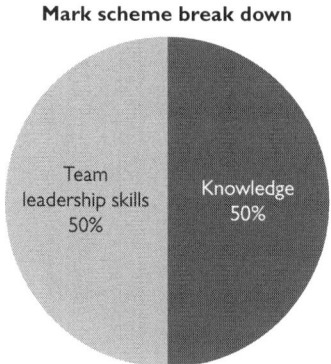

Mark scheme break down

Instructions for actor

You are a staff nurse in the ED. You know where all the equipment is kept, and can hand it to the candidate, but you don't act without being clearly instructed to do so.

Instructions for examiner

If asked by the candidate, you may give the following information:

This was a concealed pregnancy; the mother does not know how long she has been pregnant for. The baby looks nearly full term from its size.

The baby has not cried, made any noise, or breathed. It is a blue colour.

It does not respond to basic airway manoeuvres, ventilation, cardiopulmonary resuscitation (CPR), or other treatment.

A heart rate (HR) of 30–40 beats per minute (bpm) can be seen on the monitor.

You may ask the candidate what they would like to do next, but do not prompt. The candidate should be allowed to continue until the time limit of the station. The baby can be assumed to weigh 3.5 kg.

Equipment required

Paediatric resuscitation equipment
Model neonate/doll
Towel/sheet/pillow case
Baby hat
Umbilical catheters
Scalpel
Defibrillator/cardiac monitoring should be set up to show an HR of 30–40 bpm

Curriculum mapping

Sections of the CEM (2010) curriculum relevant to this question include the following.

Common competencies

CC1 History taking
CC2 Clinical examination
CC3 Therapeutics and safe prescribing
CC4 Time management and decision-making
CC5 Decision-making and clinical reasoning
CC6 Patient as the central focus of care
CC7 Prioritization of patient safety in clinical practice
CC8 Team work and patient safety
CC10 Infection control
CC12 Relationship with patients and communication
CC15 Communication with colleagues and cooperation

ACCS Major presentations CT1&2

CMP2 Cardiac arrest

CT3 Acute presentations

C3AP6 Emergency airway care

Paediatric CT3 competencies

PAP13 Neonatal presentations
PMP3 Cardiac arrest

Guidelines available

http://www.resus.org.uk/pages/nlsalgo.pdf

Mark scheme

Calls for neonatal resuscitation team	2
Takes a quick history:	
• Full term?	1
• Clear amniotic fluid?	1
• Has baby breathed/cried yet?	1
Dries baby	2
Wraps baby (towel/sheet/pillow case)	2
Positions baby correctly on bed/resuscitaire	1
Clears airway	2
During assessment/resuscitation puts head in neutral position	1
Dries, stimulates, and repositions	1
Assesses baby:	
• Breathing—rate and quality	1

Continued

Question 2 Neonatal resuscitation

Continued

• HR—fast, slow, absent, **by auscultation**	1
• Colour and tone	1
Gives 5 inflation breaths (2 points for good technique)	2
Reassesses breathing and HR after inflation breaths	1
Gives ventilation (2 for good technique)	2
Mentions rate of 30–40 per minute	1
Gives chest compressions (score 2 for good technique including rate of 100 per minute)	2
Ensures ratio of 1 breath to 3 compressions	1
Reassesses and recognizes no response to resuscitation	1
Mentions/undertakes intubation	2
Mentions/undertakes umbilical venous access	2
Mentions/gives adrenaline at dose of 0.1 ml/kg of 1/10,000 (0.35 ml for this 3.5-kg baby)	2
Considers/gives 10% dextrose at dose of 2.5 ml/kg (8.75 ml for this 3.5-kg baby)	1
Considers/gives bicarbonate at dose of 1–2 mmol (2–4 ml)/kg of 4.2% bicarbonate (3.5–7 ml for this 3.5-kg baby)	1
Considers/gives fluid	1
Demonstrates systematic, organized approach	2
Global score from examiner	5
Global score from actor	5
Total	**48**

Question 3 Cardiovascular examination

Instructions for candidate
This 78-year-old gentleman has attended the ED with a 2-hour history of chest pain which has now settled. Please examine his cardiovascular system, and describe your findings to the examiner.

Mark scheme break down

- Communication skills 20%
- Knowledge 80%

Instructions for actor
Please allow the patient to examine you. Do not prompt them, e.g. by changing position. Please make it clear if they cause you any discomfort.

Instructions for examiner
Allow the candidate to examine the patient. Two minutes before the end, stop them, and instruct them to describe their examination findings. Do not prompt the candidate in any other way.

Equipment required
None

Curriculum mapping
Sections of the CEM (2010) curriculum relevant to this question include the following.

Common competencies
CC2 Clinical examination
CC4 Time management and decision-making
CC6 Patient as the central focus of care
CC7 Prioritization of patient safety in clinical practice
CC12 Relationship with patients and communication
CC15 Communication with colleagues and cooperation

ACCS Acute presentations CT1&2
CAP7 Chest pain
CAP23 Pain management

Question 3 Cardiovascular examination

Mark scheme

Introduces self	1
Washes hands	1
Offers chaperone	1
Positions patient sitting at a 45-degree angle	1
Adequately exposes patient's chest and abdomen, whilst considering patient's dignity	1
Carries out general inspection:	3
• Comments that patient appears well	
• Looks for clues such as oxygen	
• Comments on patient's position	
• Pallor	
Inspects hands:	3
• Pallor, anaemia	
• Peripheral cyanosis	
• General perfusion including capillary refill time (CRT)	
• Clubbing	
• Signs of infective endocarditis (splinter haemorrhages)	
• Nicotine staining	
Palpates radial/brachial pulse:	1
• Measures rate	1
• Comments on characteristics	1
• Compares right and left for delay and asymmetry	1
Assesses jugular venous pressure (JVP)	1
Inspects face:	3
• Pallor	
• Central cyanosis	
• Xanthalasmata	
• Corneal arcus	
• Malar flush	
Inspects the precordium:	2
• Scars	
• Visible pulsations	
Palpates for heaves and thrills	1
Auscultates in correct positions:	
• Apex: 5th intercostal space, anterior/mid-axillary line	1
• Pulmonary valve: left sternal edge, 2nd–4th intercostal space	1
• Aortic valve: right sternal edge, 2nd–4th intercostal space	1
• Tricuspid valve: left sternal edge, 5th–6th intercostal space	1
• Mitral valve: mid-clavicular line, 5th–6th intercostal space	1

Continued

Self-Assessment for the MCEM Part C

Continued

Manoeuvres to improve auscultation:	
• Positions patient on left side and listens with bell in expiration	1
• Sits patient forwards and listens with diaphragm in expiration	1
Auscultates lung bases	1
Looks for sacral oedema	1
Looks for ankle oedema	1
Examines abdomen:	1
• Hepatomegaly	
• Palpable aneurysms	
• Femoral pulses	
Demonstrates systematic, organized approach	2
Concisely and correctly summarizes findings	5
Thanks patient	1
Global score from examiner	5
Global score from actor	5
Total	**51**

Question 4 Catheterization

Instructions for candidate

A 70-year-old man attends the ED with a 24-hour history of being unable to pass urine. He is very uncomfortable. He has been told by his General Practitioner (GP) that he has an enlarged prostate, but has never had this problem before. Please catheterize the patient using the equipment provided.

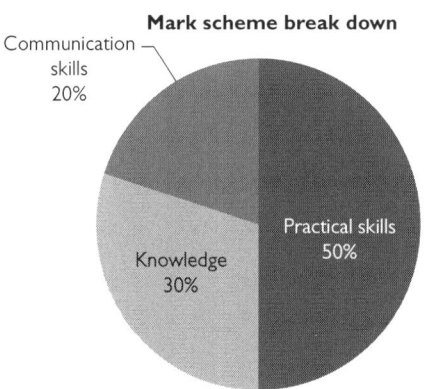

Instructions for examiner

Observation only.

Equipment required

'Model' male pelvis for catheterization
Gloves
Apron
Choice of catheters
Syringes
Anaesthetic gel
Sterile saline
Catheter drainage bag
Cleaning pack

Curriculum mapping

Sections of the CEM (2010) curriculum relevant to this question include the following.

Common competencies

CC4 Time management and decision-making
CC6 Patient as the central focus of care
CC10 Infection control
CC12 Relationship with patients and communication
CC18 Valid consent

ACCS Acute presentations CT1&2
CAP1 Abdominal pain
CAP22 Oliguric patient
CAP23 Pain management

CT3 Acute presentations
C3AP9 Urinary retention

Mark scheme

Introduces self	1
Confirms identity of patient	1
Offers chaperone	1
Obtains verbal consent	2
Washes hands	1
Maintains aseptic technique throughout	1
Adequately cleans penis	1
Uses drapes to create aseptic field	1
Uses anaesthetic gel	1
Inserts catheter to correct distance	1
Waits for urinary flow to confirm position	1
Inflates balloon correctly	1
Replaces foreskin	1
Connects catheter bag	1
Covers patient/maintains dignity	1
Tidies away equipment	1
Washes hands afterwards	1
Offers reassuring explanation to patient throughout	2
Offers discharge advice to patient:	
• Follow-up with urology arranged	1
• Catheter care pack provided	1
Global score from examiner	5
Global score from actor	5
Total	**32**

Question 5 Pulled elbow

Instructions for candidate

You have been asked to speak to the mother of a 2-year-old patient (Amy) who attended the ED with a pulled elbow. The injury happened when the child was being lifted up a step, and has been treated by the triage nurse. However, the child's mother would like an explanation about what has happened, and would like an X-ray to be taken to make sure there is no break.

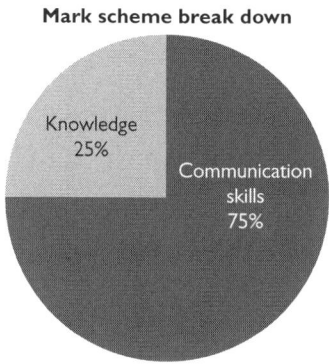

Mark scheme break down

Instructions for actor

You are the mother of a toddler, Amy. When you were helping Amy up a step into your house, she cried out, and has seemed reluctant to use her left arm ever since. You were worried she had broken something, so brought her to hospital. The triage nurse took a history about what had happened, and then moved Amy's arm about, which seemed to sort out the problem, and Amy is back to normal. The triage nurse told you 'it's just a pulled elbow', but you would like a more thorough explanation. If given the chance you should ask the following questions:

Is anything broken?
Does it need an X-ray?
Is it my fault?
Will it happen again?
Will her bones grow normally after this injury?

You accept the explanation given and accept the candidate's advice.

Instructions for examiner

Observation only.

Equipment required

None

Curriculum mapping

Sections of the CEM (2010) curriculum relevant to this question include the following.

Common competencies

CC1 History taking
CC4 Time management and decision-making

CC5 Decision-making and clinical reasoning
CC6 Patient as the central focus of care
CC7 Prioritization of patient safety in clinical practice
CC12 Relationship with patients and communication
CC16 Health promotion and public health

Paediatric CT3 competencies

PAP6 Concerning presentations
PAP15 Pain in children
PAP17 Painful limbs—traumatic

Mark scheme

Introduces self	1
Confirms Amy's mother's identity	2
Confirms history of injury	1
Confirms understanding so far	2
Accurately describes condition	3
Advises against X-ray and provides explanation	2
Invites questions	1
Deals adequately with concerns	3
Thanks mother	1
Reassures	2
Uses open and closed questioning style	2
Shows non-verbal communication skills	2
Global score from examiner	5
Global score from actor	5
Total	**32**

Question 6 Chest aspiration

Instructions for candidate
This patient has had his first ever left-sided spontaneous pneumothorax. His chest X-ray (CXR) shows that the pneumothorax involves about 50% of the left hemithorax. The patient is comfortable. He has no medical problems. Please explain the diagnosis and treatment to the patient, and demonstrate how you would treat the condition using the actor provided. **Do not** actually perform any procedures on the patient, but demonstrate to the examiner.

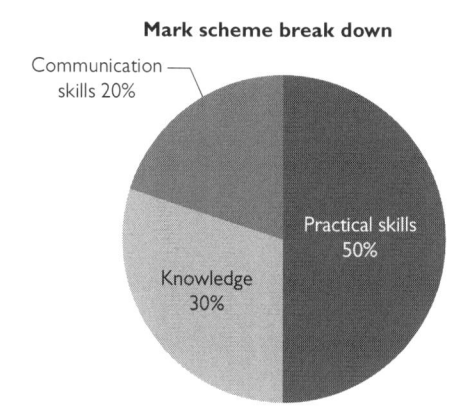

Mark scheme break down
- Communication skills 20%
- Practical skills 50%
- Knowledge 30%

Instructions for actor
You are a young man, who is normally fit and well. You have no medical problems. You had a sudden severe pain in your chest about an hour ago, but no other symptoms. You are waiting to hear the results of your X-ray, and the treatment you need. You are worried that there might be something painful involved, but when the doctor explains it, you agree to the procedure.

Instructions for examiner
Observational role but make sure the candidate does not actually perform the procedure on the patient. Rather than simply describing the procedure, you can prompt the candidate to show what they mean on the patient, e.g. landmarks.

Equipment required
Appropriate CXR
Selection of needles and syringes
Selection of IV cannulae
Liquid to simulate local anaesthetic
Three-way tap
Cleaning solution
Gauze swabs
Dressings

Curriculum mapping
Sections of the CEM (2010) curriculum relevant to this question include the following.

Common competencies

CC1 History taking
CC2 Clinical examination
CC3 Therapeutics and safe prescribing
CC4 Time management and decision-making
CC5 Decision-making and clinical reasoning
CC6 Patient as the central focus of care
CC7 Prioritization of patient safety in clinical practice
CC8 Team work and patient safety
CC9 Principles of safety and quality improvement
CC10 Infection control
CC12 Relationship with patients and communication
CC15 Communication with colleagues and cooperation
CC18 Valid consent

ACCS Acute presentations CT1&2

CAP6 Breathlessness
CAP7 Chest pain
CAP9 Cough
CAP23 Pain management

Guidelines available

http://www.brit-thoracic.org.uk/guidelines/pleuraldiseaseguidelines/

Mark scheme

Introduces self	1
Gives clear explanation of diagnosis to patient	2
Shows patient CXR	1
Checks/confirms side of pneumothorax—either with patient or using X-ray	1
Gives clear explanation of procedure to patient	2
Addresses patient's concerns	2
Invites questions	1
Prepares for procedure:	
• Semi-reclined	1
• Electrocardiogram (ECG), blood pressure (BP), and saturations monitoring in place	1
Correctly identifies anatomical landmarks:	
• Second intercostal space	1
• Mid-clavicular line	1
• Injection site immediately superior to rib	1
Uses aseptic technique throughout	1
Describes/demonstrates local anaesthetic (1% plain lignocaine 3 ml/kg to max 200 mg)	1
Describes/demonstrates passing needle correctly	1
Describes/demonstrates aspirating air correctly	1

Continued

Question 6 Chest aspiration

Continued

Communicates with patient throughout	2
Explains discharge advice:	
• Repeat CXR at 4–6 weeks in respiratory clinic	1
• Re-attend ED if pain or shortness of breath (SOB) worsens	1
• Avoid flying for 6 weeks +/− until seen in respiratory clinic	1
• Avoid scuba-diving permanently	1
Demonstrates systematic, organized approach	2
Global score from examiner	5
Global score from actor	5
Total	**37**

Question 7 Returning traveller

Instructions for candidate
Please take a history from this university student who attends the ED with a 5-day history of fever and feeling generally unwell.

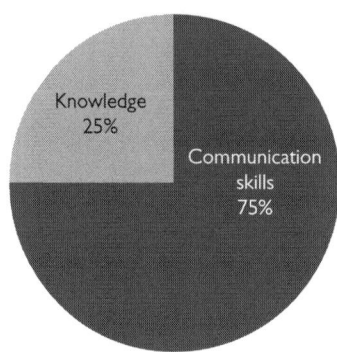

Mark scheme break down

- Knowledge 25%
- Communication skills 75%

Instructions for actor
You are a student in your early 20s. You have been feeling unwell for about 5 days. You have had intermittent fevers and shivers, vomiting, and diarrhoea. You have lost your appetite and feel very weak. You have had mild abdominal pain and aching limbs. You haven't been drinking much because you feel sick, and have noticed your urine is darker than normal. You have no other symptoms.

You have spent the summer working in Tanzania on a charity project near Dar Es Salaam for 3 months. You have taken antimalarials for most of the time, but ran out at the end because you decided to stay on an extra 2 weeks. You were based mostly in the city, but went on several trips into rural areas. You were bitten by mosquitoes frequently, even though you used repellent and nets. Whilst in Tanzania you had sex with another volunteer worker from Europe, but you always used condoms. You sometimes smoke cannabis but use no other drugs. You rarely drink alcohol. (If a female actor) Your last period was 2 weeks ago.

Before travelling, you went to the student health service and had all the vaccinations that they advised you to have, but you're not sure what they were. In the past year, you have also been on holiday to France at Christmas. Before that, you have travelled to Europe several times. You have no medical problems and are not on any medication. You are a French language student. You have no family history.

Instructions for examiner
Observation only.

Equipment required
None

Curriculum mapping
Sections of the CEM (2010) curriculum relevant to this question include the following.

Question 7 Returning traveller

Common competencies

CC1 History taking
CC5 Decision-making and clinical reasoning
CC6 Patient as the central focus of care
CC10 Infection control
CC11 Management of long-term conditions and promoting patient self-care
CC12 Relationship with patients and communication

ACCS Major presentations CT1&2

CMP4 Septic patient

ACCS Acute presentations CT1&2

CAP11 Diarrhoea
CAP14 Fever
CAP17 Headache
CAP23 Pain management
CAP36 Vomiting and nausea

Mark scheme

Introduces self	1
Establishes reason for attendance	2
Obtains thorough history of presenting complaint:	
• Clarifies nature of symptoms	1
• Clarifies duration of symptoms	1
Asks about specific travelling history (areas and timing of travel)	3
Asks about key symptoms in detail:	
• Abdominal pain	1
• Diarrhoea	1
• Headache	1
Asks about risk factors for malaria, e.g. antimalarials, nets	3
Establishes that antimalarials were not taken consistently	2
Asks about sexual history	2
Obtains immunization history	2
Asks about alcohol history	2
Asks about drug use	2
Asks about medications	1
Obtains past medical history	1
Summarizes history	3
Advises course of action to include investigations for malaria, including thick and thin films	2
Global score from examiner	5
Global score from actor	5
Total	**42**

Question 8 Paronychia

Instructions for candidate
This patient attends with paronychia. Please explain how you would like to treat it, and demonstrate to the examiner how you would do this (**do not** actually perform a procedure on the patient).

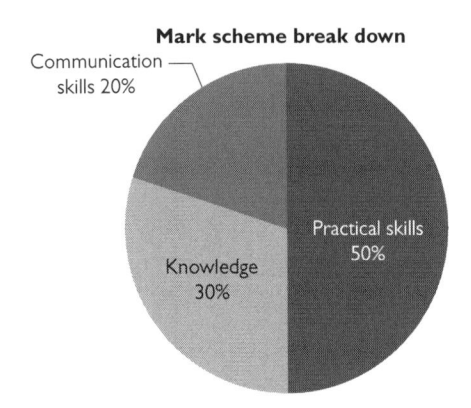

Mark scheme break down
- Communication skills 20%
- Knowledge 30%
- Practical skills 50%

Instructions for actor
You have a small abscess on the side of one of your fingernails which is very painful. You think it started when you ripped your fingernail on a kitchen door 2 days ago. You would like to have it sorted out, and go along with whatever the doctor recommends.

Instructions for examiner
Allow the candidate to explain the procedure to the candidate. You may prompt them to demonstrate the technique to move the candidate on to this part of the station.

Equipment required
Selection of needles and syringes
Liquid to simulate local anaesthetic
Cleaning solution
Gauze swabs
Scalpel
Dressings

Curriculum mapping
Sections of the CEM (2010) curriculum relevant to this question include the following.

Common competencies

CC1 History taking
CC2 Clinical examination
CC3 Therapeutics and safe prescribing
CC4 Time management and decision-making
CC5 Decision-making and clinical reasoning
CC6 Patient as the central focus of care

Question 8 Paronychia

CC7 Prioritization of patient safety in clinical practice
CC10 Infection control
CC12 Relationship with patients and communication

ACCS Acute presentations CT1&2

CAP20 Limb pain and swelling—atraumatic
CAP23 Pain management
CAP33 Traumatic limb and joint injuries
CAP38 Wound assessment and management

Mark scheme

Introduces self	1
Explains diagnosis	2
Explains treatment including procedure	2
Reassures with explanation	2
Invites questions	2
Washes hands	1
Puts on gloves	1
Uses aseptic technique	1
Offers option of ring block to patient:	
• Two or three injection sites at base of finger	1
• Local anaesthetic to provide anaesthesia	1
• Dose of 1% plain lignocaine, maximum 3 ml/kg to max 200 mg	1
• Suggest total of approximately 5 ml volume	1
Incises into paronychia using scalpel	2
Expresses pus	1
Leaves wound open	1
Applies dressing	1
Offers advice for follow-up/when to seek help	1
Global score from examiner	5
Global score from actor	5
Total	**32**

Question 9 Breaking bad news 1

Instructions for candidate
You have been looking after an 89-year-old woman, Mrs Smith, who collapsed suddenly at home and has been unconscious ever since. She has had a computerized tomography (CT) scan, which shows a large intracranial bleed. You have discussed her with the neurosurgical consultant, who does not want to operate because of the poor prognosis. Her daughter has just arrived at the hospital and has been told by the ED receptionist that her mother is in resus. You should explain to her daughter what has happened, and answer any questions she has.

Mark scheme break down

- Knowledge 25%
- Communication skills 75%

Instructions for actor
You are the daughter of Mrs Smith, an elderly woman who has collapsed at home. You were phoned at work by the hospital and told to come straight in, as she is very unwell. You have not been told anything else.

Until today, your mother was living by herself in her own flat, and had a good quality of life. She has been told she has osteoporosis (thin bones) by the GP who started her on some tablets, and mild asthma for which she takes inhalers every now and then. She has no help around the flat, and goes out to the shops most days. She is very active, and enjoys the company of her grandchildren and great grandchildren. You would describe her as a 'fighter' and feel certain that she will survive this and recover because she has always been so healthy. If asked about her wishes, you tell the doctor that you have never talked about end-of-life decisions, but you would like everything possible done to keep her alive, even if her heart stopped beating.

If given the chance, you want to know the following:

How do you know that the prognosis is so bad?
What are the chances she will survive?
How long will it take to die?
Is this something that could have been prevented?
Can you see her?

You are very upset when the doctor explains how unwell your mother is. You go along with what the doctor says. You agree that she should not be resuscitated.

Instructions for examiner
Observation only.

Equipment required
Appropriate CT images

Question 9 Breaking bad news I

Curriculum mapping

Sections of the CEM (2010) curriculum relevant to this question include the following.

Common competencies

CC1 History taking
CC4 Time management and decision-making
CC5 Decision-making and clinical reasoning
CC6 Patient as the central focus of care
CC8 Team work and patient safety
CC13 Breaking bad news

ACCS Major presentations CT1&2

CMP6 Unconscious patient

ACCS Acute presentations CT1&2

CAP5 Blackout/collapse
CAP13 Falls
CAP18 Head injury
CAP32 Syncope and presyncope

Mark scheme

Introduces self	1
Asks for a nurse/family member to accompany them	1
Ensures bleep/mobile phone is switched off/silent	1
Ensures nurse in charge is aware of location in department	1
Checks correct identity	1
Establishes what is already known	2
Explains diagnosis clearly	2
Demonstrates CT appearance	1
Conveys poor prognosis	2
Invites questions	1
Explains poor prognosis	2
Asks about prior quality of life	2
Introduces end of life issues sensitively	2
Uses clear language such as 'death'/'dying'/'will not survive'	1
Does not indicate that family can choose to resuscitate	1
Discusses Intensive Therapy Unit (ITU)/resuscitation	3
Answers questions adequately	2
Offers that family can see patient	1
Displays appropriate use of silence	1
Has appropriate body language	1
Global score from examiner	5
Global score from actor	5
Total	**37**

Question 10 Forearm plaster

Instructions for candidate
Your patient has an undisplaced distal radial fracture. Please apply a suitable plaster and get them ready for discharge home.

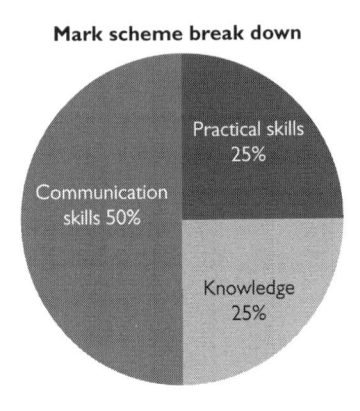

Mark scheme break down

- Practical skills 25%
- Communication skills 50%
- Knowledge 25%

Instructions for actor
You are a patient in their 60s who has recently retired. You are right-handed. You live with your partner and you are very independent. You have fallen over whilst out walking this morning. You have had an X-ray which showed a broken left wrist. The break is not too bad, but it needs to be put in plaster. Your wrist is painful, and you don't like it to be touched or moved. The candidate should apply a plaster cast to your forearm without causing you any additional pain.

You would like some painkillers to take home with you. You think you will manage fine at home, with a little help from your partner, and decline the offer of any additional help.

Instructions for examiner
Mainly observational.

When/if the candidate has completed the plaster, you may prompt them with the question 'is there anything you would like to tell the patient before sending them home?'

Equipment required
Standard plaster kit
Appropriate X-ray

Curriculum mapping
Sections of the CEM (2010) curriculum relevant to this question include the following.

Common competencies

CC2 Clinical examination
CC3 Therapeutics and safe prescribing
CC4 Time management and decision-making
CC5 Decision-making and clinical reasoning
CC6 Patient as the central focus of care
CC7 Prioritization of patient safety in clinical practice

CC8 Team work and patient safety
CC9 Principles of safety and quality improvement
CC10 Infection control
CC12 Relationship with patients and communication
CC18 Valid consent

ACCS Acute presentations CT1&2

CAP23 Pain management
CAP33 Traumatic limb and joint injuries

Mark scheme

Introduces self	1
Asks about/offers analgesia	1
Explains need for plaster	1
Demonstrates fracture on X-ray	1
Correctly positions patient	2
Measures plaster	1
Applies correct thickness of plaster	1
Applies Tubinette™/gauze layers	1
Demonstrates correct placement of plaster on arm (dorsal)	2
Secures with bandage	1
Moulds plaster around fracture site	1
Ensures no rough edges	1
Plaster covers from elbow to metacarpal-phalangeal joint (MCPJ) and checks movement	2
Checks distal neurovascular supply	1
Mentions/applies sling	1
Advises about plaster—getting wet, swelling, etc.	2
Checks how patient will manage in plaster	1
Explains how follow-up in clinic will be arranged	1
Invites questions	1
Demonstrates systematic, organized approach	2
Global score from examiner	5
Global score from actor	5
Total	**34**

Question 11 Sickle cell disease

Instructions for candidate
This patient has attended the ED with abdominal pain, by ambulance. He tells you he has sickle cell disease and frequently needs admission when he is in crisis, for IV fluids and analgesia. Please take a history from him and discuss his management with him.

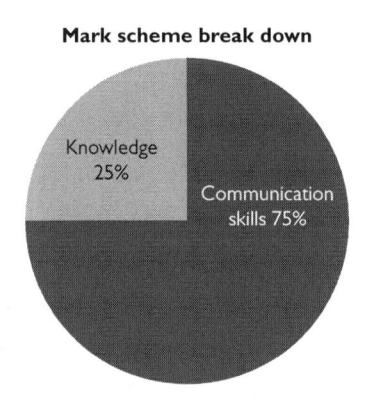

Mark scheme break down

- Knowledge 25%
- Communication skills 75%

Instructions for actor
You have a diagnosis of sickle cell disease that gives you attacks of pain in your abdomen and various other places. When these attacks happen, you need to go to hospital for painkillers and IV fluids. You have often been admitted to the haematology ward. Today, you tell the doctors, you have had 10 minutes of severe central abdominal pain, with no other symptoms. You were watching TV when it came on.

You have previously been an IV drug user, and you take methadone every day, as prescribed by your GP. You find it very difficult to manage without heroin and think that your prescribed dose of methadone is too low. When you get really desperate, you phone 999 in the hope that the paramedics or hospital staff will give you a morphine injection. You know that if you tell them you are having a sickle cell crisis, they usually take you seriously. You know that the only thing that will make you feel better is morphine. You get very angry if the doctor suggests you are not genuine or refuses to give you morphine. You threaten to report them and beg them for morphine. You refuse any other painkillers offered.

You should give the history if prompted by the candidate. Do not volunteer your history of IV drug use unless directly asked about drug use. You are reluctant to answer many questions from the candidate, because you just want to get the morphine. You try to get them to hurry up and prescribe some morphine.

Instructions for examiner
Observation only.

Equipment required
None

Curriculum mapping
Sections of the CEM (2010) curriculum relevant to this question include the following.

Question 11 Sickle cell disease

Common competencies

CC1 History taking
CC3 Therapeutics and safe prescribing
CC4 Time management and decision-making
CC5 Decision-making and clinical reasoning
CC6 Patient as the central focus of care
CC7 Prioritization of patient safety in clinical practice
CC8 Team work and patient safety
CC9 Principles of safety and quality improvement
CC11 Management of long-term conditions and promoting patient self-care
CC12 Relationship with patients and communication
CC15 Communication with colleagues and cooperation

ACCS Acute presentations CT1&2

CAP1 Abdominal pain including loin pain
CAP3 Acute back pain
CAP4 Aggressive/disturbed behaviour
CAP23 Pain management

Mark scheme

Introduces self	1
Obtains focused history of presenting complaint	4
Obtains past medical history:	
• Sickle cell	1
• Drug use	1
Asks about drug use history:	
• Drug abuse	1
• Methadone	1
Offers alternative analgesia (not morphine)	2
Does not challenge/accuse patient of drug-seeking behaviour	2
Refuses to be convinced to prescribe morphine	2
Advises about investigations needed	1
Is calm and professional throughout	2
Global score from examiner	5
Global score from actor	5
Total	**27**

Question 12 Explaining an error

Instructions for candidate
You are working in a busy ED. There are two toddlers in the department. One has a suspected pneumonia and needs a CXR. You requested it yourself, but accidentally stuck another child's name sticker on the card in error.

The other child was meant to have a wrist X-ray, but instead had a CXR. Please explain to the parents of the child who has had an unnecessary CXR what has happened, and why they need to go back to the X-ray department a second time to get the correct X-ray done.

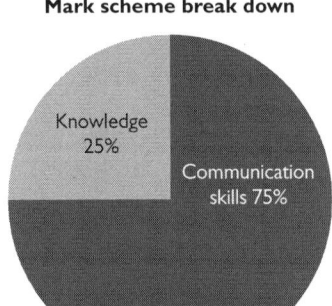

Mark scheme break down

- Knowledge 25%
- Communication skills 75%

Instructions for actors
Your child (Billy) fell over in the garden and ever since then has not been using his wrist, and his forearm looks bent out of shape. You have seen a doctor, who told you it looked broken and has sent you round for an X-ray of your child's arm. When you got to the X-ray department, Billy got very upset and started screaming, so it was difficult to hear what people were telling you to do. You had to pin him down to have an X-ray taken, and it was very upsetting for all of you.

When the candidate/doctor explains that Billy had the wrong type of X-ray, you are really upset. You think he is traumatized by the event, and you have read in a magazine that X-rays cause cancer. You want to know who is to blame and how to make a complaint. You also want to know what will happen to poor Billy now. If the candidate/doctor offers you their apologies, you accept them but still want to make a formal complaint. You want to make sure this will not happen again.

Instructions for examiner
Observation only.

Equipment required
None

Curriculum mapping
Sections of the CEM (2010) curriculum relevant to this question include the following.

Common competencies

CC6 Patient as the central focus of care
CC7 Prioritization of patient safety in clinical practice

Question 12 Explaining an error

CC12 Relationship with patients and communication
CC14 Complaints and medical error
CC18 Valid consent

Mark scheme

Introduces self	1
Checks identity	1
Tells parent that wrong X-ray was taken (CXR instead of wrist X-ray)	2
Explains honestly why it has happened—human error	2
Apologizes	2
Explains that the correct X-ray now needs to be done	1
Checks/offers additional analgesia	1
Addresses concerns adequately	2
Defuses situation	2
Is empathic throughout	2
Offers mechanism to make a complaint	2
Accepts blame/takes responsibility	2
Global score from examiner	5
Global score from actor	5
Total	**32**

Question 13 Chest pain 1

Instructions for candidate
This young person has been brought into hospital following an episode of chest pain. Please take a history and explain to the patient what you would like to do.

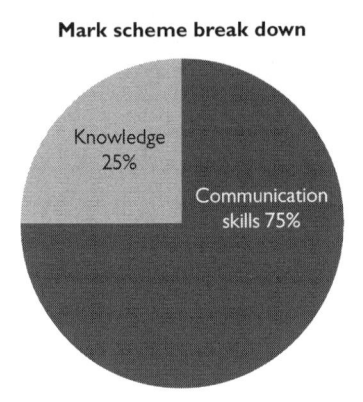

Mark scheme break down

(Pie chart: Knowledge 25%, Communication skills 75%)

Instructions for actor
You are a 24-year-old drama student. Your friends called for an ambulance this evening because you had an episode of chest pain whilst out in a nightclub. You describe the chest pain as a heavy ache across your chest, which made you feel dizzy and unwell. At the same time, you had palpitations/felt your heart racing. You were on the dance floor when the pain came on and you told a friend, who helped you to sit down and phoned 999. Your friends told you that you looked very pale. You have been out celebrating a friend's birthday and have had several shots of vodka and some cocaine. You regularly take cocaine with your group of friends when you go out at weekends. You don't drink alcohol apart from when you go out at weekends, and you don't smoke. You consider yourself very healthy—you watch what you eat and go to the gym nearly every day. You have no medical problems or family history and don't take any prescribed medications.

The paramedic gave you some oxygen to breath, and a medicine that came as a spray under your tongue, in the ambulance which made you feel better within about 5 minutes. You now feel absolutely fine and want to go home. You think the candidate is being ridiculous if they suggest you need some investigations or to stay in hospital. You have never heard about the risks of taking cocaine, and all your friends do it, so you think it is safer than drinking alcohol. You are reluctant to stay in hospital, but allow yourself to be persuaded by the candidate.

Instructions for examiner
Allow the candidate to take a history. When there are 3 minutes left in the station, if the candidate has not already done so, you may prompt them to move on to explaining to the patient what the management plan is. You should interrupt them to do this if necessary.

Equipment required
None

Curriculum mapping
Sections of the CEM (2010) curriculum relevant to this question include the following.

Question 13 Chest pain 1

Common competencies

CC1 History taking
CC2 Clinical examination
CC3 Therapeutics and safe prescribing
CC4 Time management and decision-making
CC5 Decision-making and clinical reasoning
CC6 Patient as the central focus of care
CC7 Prioritization of patient safety in clinical practice
CC8 Team work and patient safety
CC12 Relationship with patients and communication

ACCS Acute presentations CT1&2

CAP7 Chest pain
CAP23 Pain management

Mark scheme

Introduces self	1
Starts with open questions	1
Uses combination of open/closed questions to clarify points in history	1
Obtains history of presenting complaint:	
• Description of chest pain	1
• Associated features	1
• Exacerbating/relieving factors	1
• Precipitating events	1
Obtains past medical history	1
Asks about drug use	1
Asks about alcohol use	1
Asks about smoking history	1
Asks about family history	1
Explains:	
• Possible diagnosis is cocaine-related chest pain	1
• Further investigations include ECG, CXR, and cardiac enzymes	1
• Need to stay in hospital	1
• That cocaine causes vasospasm and can be dangerous	1
Invites questions	1
Closure—reviews learning with student	1
Global score from examiner	5
Global score from actor	5
Total	**28**

Question 14 ECG

Instructions for candidate
This patient has attended the ED complaining of palpitations. Please take an ECG on this patient and explain your interpretation of the ECG to the examiner.

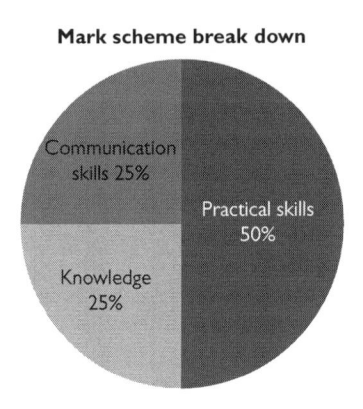

Mark scheme break down

- Communication skills 25%
- Practical skills 50%
- Knowledge 25%

Instructions for actor
Allow the candidate to take an ECG. Do not prompt the candidate, e.g. by changing position.

Instructions for examiner
Allow the candidate to take the ECG without prompting. Allow the candidate to explain the finished ECG to you. You may prompt their explanation with the following questions:

Tell me how to assess the rhythm and rate on this ECG.
Is the ECG normal or abnormal?

Equipment required
ECG machine

Curriculum mapping
Sections of the CEM (2010) curriculum relevant to this question include the following.

Common competencies

CC5 Decision-making and clinical reasoning
CC12 Relationship with patients and communication
CC18 Valid consent

ACCS Acute presentations CT1&2

CAP25 Palpitations

Question 14 ECG

Mark scheme

Introduces self	1
Provides brief explanation of procedure	2
Undresses patient	1
Maintains dignity	1
Applies chest lead stickers in correct places:	
• Lead 1 in 4th intercostal space, right sternal edge	1
• Lead 2 in 4th intercostal space, left sternal edge	1
• Lead 4 in 5th intercostal space, mid-clavicular line (at location of apex beat)	1
• Leads 3, 5, and 6 equally spaced around leads above	1
Connects leads correctly	2
Is able to produce ECG	2
Checks ECG	2
Removes stickers	1
Allows patient to get dressed	1
Thanks patient	1
Correctly interprets ECG as normal	2
Applies correct rate and rhythm	2
Global score from examiner	5
Global score from actor	5
Total	**32**

Question 15 Neurosurgical referral

Instructions for candidate

You are the registrar on nights in the ED of a small district general hospital. You are in resus with a 22-year-old man who has been assaulted on the way home from the pub 1 hour earlier. A witness described that he was punched and kicked several times in the head and was unconscious until the ambulance arrived.

When you assessed him, he had severe scalp bruising and had a Glasgow Coma Scale (GCS) of 7 (E2, V1, M4). Your anaesthetic colleague has intubated him, and a CT scan shows a small right-sided extradural haemorrhage, with no midline shift and a normal cervical spine CT. You should refer the patient to the neurosurgical registrar and arrange transfer to the neurosurgical centre in the nearest city.

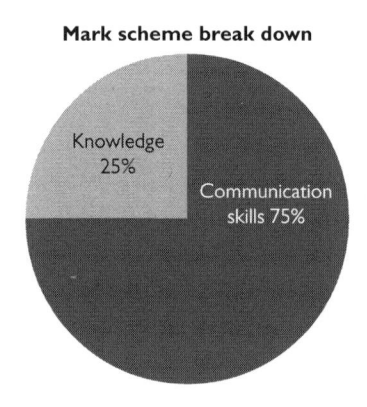

Mark scheme break down

- Knowledge 25%
- Communication skills 75%

Instructions for actor

Listen to the referral given by the candidate. Accept the referral if a clear referral is made. If not enough detail is provided, ask the following questions:

What do his injuries look like?
What was his GCS prior to intubation?
What does his CT head scan show?
Who is going to come with him to the neurosurgical centre?
If asked, instruct the candidate to transfer the patient to the neurosurgical ITU, not to theatre.

Instructions for examiner

Observation only.

Equipment required

Instructions for candidate should be available during the station
Telephone
Paper and pen
Relevant CT images

Curriculum mapping

Sections of the CEM (2010) curriculum relevant to this question include the following.

Question 15 Neurosurgical referral

Common competencies

CC4 Time management and decision-making
CC5 Decision-making and clinical reasoning
CC6 Patient as the central focus of care
CC7 Prioritization of patient safety in clinical practice
CC8 Team work and patient safety
CC15 Communication with colleagues and cooperation

ACCS Major presentations CT1&2

CMP3 Major trauma
CMP6 Unconscious patient

ACCS Acute presentations CT1&2

CAP18 Head injury

Mark scheme

Introduces self	2
Checks speaking with neurosurgical registrar	2
Confirms best way to contact neurosurgical registrar	1
States clearly that patient needs to be transferred	2
Obtains a brief history	2
Includes CT diagnosis in brief history	2
Describes GCS in brief history	2
Is aware of correct details in history when prompted	2
Makes it clear that patient is intubated	2
Makes it clear that this patient will have an anaesthetic/ED doctor to transfer them	1
Asks exactly where to transfer patient within hospital	2
Confirms bed available	2
Asks if anything else is required prior to transfer	2
Confirms will arrange ambulance urgently	2
Confirms they will contact again when patient is on the way to let them know	1
Global score from examiner	5
Global score from actor	5
Total	**37**

Question 16 Psychiatry

Instructions for candidate
Please take a history from this patient who has been brought in by ambulance after she was found acting strangely in the supermarket.

Mark scheme break down

- Knowledge 25%
- Communication skills 75%

Instructions for actor
You have been brought into hospital by ambulance from the supermarket where you were doing your weekly shopping. You were trying to hide from the closed circuit television (CCTV) cameras in the shop, because you know that the government uses the cameras to spy on you. Someone in the shop thought you were acting strangely and called an ambulance.

The government has been keeping tabs on you for a while. You think it started when you were late in paying your TV licence; since then, they have taken over your TV and use it to send you messages that they are watching you. You are reluctant to leave the house because you think there are government spies around. You have blacked out the windows in your house so they can't see in. You have cut off your phone line, electricity, and gas so the government can't monitor you. You aren't seeing things or hearing things, but you think that the TV is talking at you, and that adverts in the street are trying to communicate messages from the government to you.

You have no medical problems but previously have been an inpatient in a mental hospital, about 20 years ago. You're not sure what the problem was then, and you are supposed to take tablets and see your Community Psychiatric Nurse (CPN) regularly. You have stopped taking the tablets in case they are poisoned by the government and avoided contact with your CPN in case he is a spy. You have no insight into your mental health problems. You are not distressed or suicidal. You do not want help and would like to go home as soon as possible.

Instructions for examiner
Observation only.

Equipment required
None

Curriculum mapping
Sections of the CEM (2010) curriculum relevant to this question include the following.

Common competencies

CC1 History taking
CC2 Clinical examination
CC4 Time management and decision-making
CC5 Decision-making and clinical reasoning
CC6 Patient as the central focus of care
CC7 Prioritization of patient safety in clinical practice
CC8 Team work and patient safety
CC12 Relationship with patients and communication

ACCS Acute presentations CT1&2

CAP4 Aggressive/disturbed behaviour
CAP8 Confusion, acute/delirium
CAP30 Mental health

Mark scheme

Introduces self	1
Uses open questions to begin consultation	1
Uses the structure of the mental state examination using the areas below:	
• Appearance: comments on patient's appearance	1
• Behaviour: asks about or comments on behaviour	1
• Mood and affect:	
♦ Asks about mood	1
♦ Asks about symptoms of depression—libido, early morning wakening, poor appetite, etc.	1
• Speech: comments on patient's speech	1
• Thought process: comments on patient's speech (as a marker of thought process)	1
• Thought content: asks about delusions, preoccupations, overvalued ideas, obsessions	2
• Perception: asks about sensory experiences	1
• Cognition: brief assessment of cognition	1
• Insight: assessment of insight	1
Makes a brief assessment of suicide/self-harm risk	1
Asks about alcohol history	1
Asks about drug history	1
Asks about social support—friends and family	1
Obtains marital history	1
Obtains occupational history	1
Obtains past medial history	1
Obtains past psychiatric history	1
Advises patient needs mental health referral	1
Invites questions	1
Global score from examiner	5
Global score from actor	5
Total	**34**

Station 17 Knee joint aspiration

Instructions for candidate

Your consultant has asked you to aspirate the knee of a patient with a large tense atraumatic effusion. The patient is systemically well. The patient has already been consented for the procedure by your consultant. Please demonstrate the correct technique for aspiration.

Mark scheme break down
- Communication skills 20%
- Knowledge 30%
- Practical skills 50%

Instructions for examiner

Observation only.

Please note, if it is not possible to obtain a 'model' for this station, the candidate could 'talk through' the procedure, using the equipment listed, in order to practise the station.

Equipment required

'Model' knee suitable for aspiration
Appropriate X-ray—right knee effusion
Aspiration kit:

- Trolley
- Gloves
- Surgical gowns
- Surgical eye protectors/goggles
- Equipment for hand washing
- Sterile drapes
- Selection of needles/cannulae and syringes
- Three-way tape
- Local anaesthetic—lignocaine, bupivicaine
- Universal collection pots
- Chlorhexidine or similar
- Scissors
- Dressing
- Tape
- Pillow

Curriculum mapping

Sections of the CEM (2010) curriculum relevant to this question include the following.

Question 17 Knee joint aspiration

Common competencies

CC2 Clinical examination
CC3 Therapeutics and safe prescribing
CC5 Decision-making and clinical reasoning
CC6 Patient as the central focus of care
CC7 Prioritization of patient safety in clinical practice
CC10 Infection control
CC12 Relationship with patients and communication
CC15 Communication with colleagues and cooperation
CC18 Valid consent

ACCS Acute presentations CT1&2

CAP23 Pain management
CAP33 Traumatic limb and joint injuries

Mark scheme

Introduces self	1
Explains diagnosis—knee effusion +/− demonstrates X-ray	1
Explains need for aspiration—pain relief and diagnostic measure	1
Checks patient is comfortable/appropriate analgesia	1
Checks side of effusion—e.g. asks to see X-ray, confirms with patient	1
Checks patient understands procedure (patient has already been consented so is therefore aware of what is involved)	1
Prepares equipment adequately using sterile technique	2
Washes hands	1
Positions patient correctly (semireclined, right leg flexed at 90°, resting on pillow)	1
Describes appropriate approach—aim for suprapatella pouch—lateral approach—area where effusion easily palpable	1
Inserts local anaesthetic—correct choice and dose (1% plain lignocaine 3 ml/kg) and checks it has worked before starting (can use this needle to also confirm diagnosis)	2
Uses appropriate needle/cannula to perform aspiration—three-way tap and aspiration using 20-ml syringe	2
Collects sample of aspirate (should be told that it is gelatinous blood-stained fluid—not pus)	1
Comments on tests to request:	
• Cell count for white blood cells (WBCs), microscopy for organisms, urate crystals—negatively birefringent in gout	2
Considers infiltrating joint with bupivicaine for analgesia	1
Provides dressing	1
Suggests appropriate management plan for gout—non-steroidal anti-inflammatory drugs (NSAIDs) + GP follow-up	1
Communicates well with patient throughout	2
Maintains safe practice throughout—minimizes risk of personal injury	2
Global score from examiner	5
Total	**35**

Question 18 Auroscopy

Instructions for candidate

Please teach this final-year medical student how to use an auroscope/otoscope.

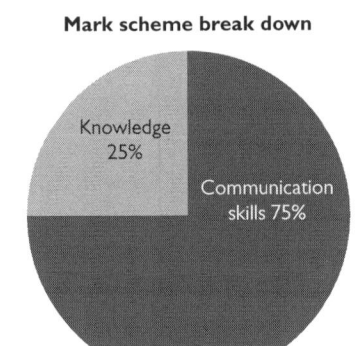

Mark scheme break down

- Knowledge 25%
- Communication skills 75%

Instructions for actor

You are a final-year medical student. You have seen auroscope (otoscope) used but have never tried to use it yourself. Do what the candidate says but don't show any initiative or do anything that they did not show you. When you are given the chance to try the technique yourself, make sure that you forget to position the pinna correctly—the candidate should correct you.

If given the chance to ask questions, ask either 'What sort of things can you diagnose from looking in someone's ears?' or 'Do you do it the same in children?', depending on what the candidate has covered in their explanation.

Instructions for examiner

Observation only.

Equipment required

Otoscope
Simulated patient (model or actor)

Curriculum mapping

Sections of the CEM (2010) curriculum relevant to this question include the following.

Common competencies

CC5 Decision-making and clinical reasoning
CC6 Patient as the central focus of care
CC15 Communication with colleagues and cooperation

ACCS Acute presentations CT1&2

CAP18 Head injury
CAP24 Painful ear

Question 18 Auroscopy

Mark scheme

Introduces self	1
Establishes entry knowledge	1
Establishes good rapport	1
Introduces topic and aim and teaching session	1
Explains equipment:	
• Light	1
• Disposable attachment	1
Prepares patient:	
• Explains procedure	1
• Ensures comfortable position	1
• Traction of patient ear/pinna	1
Explains and demonstrates technique:	
• Correctly holds auroscope	1
• Checks light working	1
• Inspects external ear	1
• Comments on internal structures including canal and tympanic membrane	1
Allows student to try technique	1
Corrects student's technique	1
Invites questions	1
Encourages practice/suggests ways to gain experience	2
Summarizes	1
Global score from examiner	5
Global score from actor	5
Total	**29**

Question 19 Shoulder examination

Instructions for candidate
This patient has fallen off their bike earlier today. He is complaining of pain in his right shoulder. Please examine his shoulder and then explain to the patient what you would like to do next.

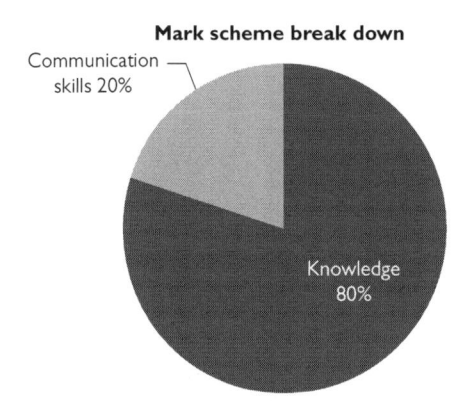

Mark scheme break down

- Communication skills 20%
- Knowledge 80%

Instructions for actor
You are a right-handed history student who has fallen off their bike earlier today. You landed on your left shoulder and, since then, it has been painful. You can't lift your arm in the air, and there is a tender lump at the end of your collar bone, where it meets the shoulder (acromioclavicular joint (ACJ)). You can do all of the movements that the candidate asks you to do, but it is very painful to do so. When the candidate presses on the end of your collar bone, it is really painful.

You have not yet had an X-ray, but you have been seen by a nurse who gave you some painkillers which have helped with the pain. You are worried that you have broken your collar bone, because you are a keen mountain biker and want to get back to normal as soon as possible.

Instructions for examiner
Observation only.

Equipment required
None

Curriculum mapping
Sections of the CEM (2010) curriculum relevant to this question include the following.

Common competencies

CC2 Clinical examination
CC5 Decision-making and clinical reasoning

ACCS Acute presentations CT1&2

CAP23 Pain management
CAP33 Traumatic limb and joint injuries

Question 19 Shoulder examination

Mark scheme

Introduces self	1
Washes hands	1
Checks analgesia given/offers analgesia	1
Asks patient to undress	1
Inspects for:	
• Signs of trauma such as bruises, swelling, deformities	1
• Scars	1
• Erythema	1
• Muscle wasting	1
• Inspects from front and behind	1
Palpates for bony tenderness, heat, and crepitus:	
• Sternoclavicular joint	1
• Clavicle	1
• ACJ	1
• Head of humerus	1
• Neck of humerus	1
• Spine of scapula	1
Checks movements:	
• Painful arc/abduction/adduction	1
• Flexion/extension	1
• Internal/external rotation	1
• Active and resisted movements tested	1
Checks for resisted movements of rotator cuff	1
Carries out instability tests:	
• Apprehension test	1
• Inspection for superior sulcus	1
Carries out impingement tests	1
Suggests or does neurovascular examination	1
Suggests or does examination of cervical spine	1
Ensures patient is dressed and comfortable	1
Thanks patient	1
Suggests ACJ problem	1
Suggests broad arm sling	1
Suggests X-ray and review	1
Demonstrates systematic, organized approach	2
Global score from examiner	5
Global score from actor	5
Total	**39**

Question 20 Overdose

Instructions for candidate
The patient has attended the ED after taking an overdose of 8 ibuprofen 6 hours ago. His blood tests, done by the triage nurse, are normal, including paracetamol and salicylate levels. Please take a history from the patient.

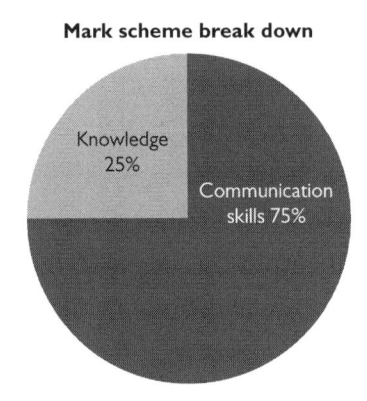

Mark scheme break down

- Knowledge 25%
- Communication skills 75%

Instructions for actor
You have taken an overdose because you want to die. You are a middle-aged man who has recently separated from his wife after finding out that she had been having an affair. She has moved out of the family home that you shared for 20 years. Your children are grown up and are at university. You were made redundant last year from your job as a bus driver. You have some friends nearby, who are very supportive, but socializing tends to centre on your local pub, and you have been drinking every day recently to 'forget' what is going on. You can't remember the last day you didn't have a drink and get shaky if you don't have any alcohol by lunchtime. Since you were made redundant, you have been struggling to pay the mortgage, but no-one knows this.

You think that if you go home, you would eventually try to kill yourself again, but have no immediate plans to do so. You took the tablets today after getting drunk and realizing you have nothing left to live for. You now feel a bit silly about it, but still very low. You realized you had done something dangerous, so came to hospital to get checked over. You thought that the amount of ibuprofen taken could kill you. You haven't seen your doctor for years and have no medical problems that you know of.

Instructions for examiner
Observation only.

Equipment required
None

Curriculum mapping
Sections of the CEM (2010) curriculum relevant to this question include the following.

Common competencies
CC1 History taking
CC2 Clinical examination
CC3 Therapeutics and safe prescribing
CC4 Time management and decision-making
CC5 Decision-making and clinical reasoning

CC6 Patient as the central focus of care
CC7 Prioritization of patient safety in clinical practice
CC9 Principles of safety and quality improvement
CC10 Infection control
CC12 Relationship with patients and communication

ACCS Acute presentations CT1&2

CAP27 Poisoning
CAP30 Mental health

Guidelines available

http://publications.nice.org.uk/self-harm-cg16

Mark scheme

Introduces self	1
Establishes tablets taken and timing	1
Explains blood test ok	1
Asks reason for overdose	1
Establishes circumstances—alcohol, reasons, note, etc.	2
Asks reason for discovery/seeking help	1
Undertakes suicide risk assessment using SADPERSONS scale:	10 total for this section
S: Male sex	
A: Older age	
D: Depression	
P: Previous attempt	
E: Ethanol or drug abuse	
R: Rational thinking loss	
S: Social supports lacking	
O: Organized plan	
N: No spouse	
S: Sickness	
Uses results of SADPERSONS score to categorize risk based on the following:	2
0–4 Low	
5–6 Medium	
7–10 High	
Obtains medication history	1
Asks about drug use	1
Obtains past medical history	1
Obtains past psychiatric history	1
Advises patient they need mental health referral	1
Invites questions	1
Global score from examiner	5
Global score from actor	5
Total	**35**

Question 21 Suturing

Instructions for candidate
This patient has cut their right forearm on a broken piece of glass. They have a linear 2-cm laceration on their dorsal forearm. They have had an X-ray which shows no foreign body in the wound, and they are neurovascularly intact. Please suture the wound, using the equipment provided.

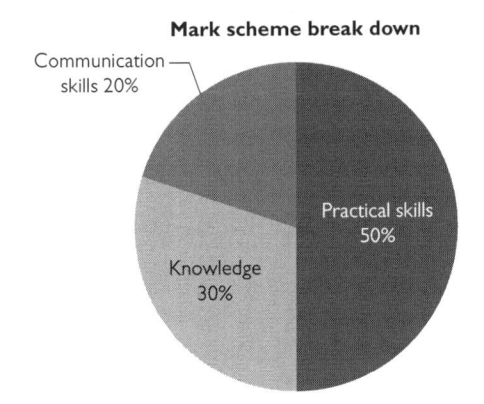

Mark scheme break down
- Communication skills 20%
- Knowledge 30%
- Practical skills 50%

Instructions for actor
You are a right-handed builder and are worried that you won't be able to work with this injury. You are up to date with your tetanus, have no medical problems, and no allergies.

Instructions for examiner
Observation only.
   Please ensure that the candidate uses the model skin provided, and does not attempt to suture the actor.

Equipment required
Appropriate forearm X-ray showing no foreign body
Simulated skin
Selection of sutures
Suture kit (needle holder, toothed forceps, non-toothed forceps, suture scissors)
Gauze
Simulated local anaesthetic, in syringe with needle
Sterile and non-sterile gloves in selection of sizes

Curriculum mapping
Sections of the CEM (2010) curriculum relevant to this question include the following.

Common competencies

CC2 Clinical examination
CC3 Therapeutics and safe prescribing
CC5 Decision-making and clinical reasoning
CC6 Patient as the central focus of care

Question 21 Suturing

CC10 Infection control
CC12 Relationship with patients and communication

ACCS Acute presentations CT1&2

CAP23 Pain management
CAP33 Traumatic limb and joint injuries
CAP38 Wound assessment and management

Mark scheme

Introduces self	1
Washes hands	1
Checks if analgesia given/required	1
Asks patient about status and date of last tetanus vaccination	1
Explains procedure	2
Suggests local anaesthetic and explains which and dose regime (lignocaine 3 mg/kg)	1
Allows time to work/checks anaesthesia	1
Selects correct suture (4.0 non-absorbable)	1
Applies thorough saline lavage	1
Carries out suturing correctly:	
• Appropriate suture placement/needle positioning	1
• No touch technique	1
• Toothed forceps used	1
• Instrument or hand tie using sterile technique	1
• Cuts sutures to appropriate length	1
• Safe technique—thorough avoidance of risks of needle-stick injury	1
• Achieves adequate closure	1
• Minus two marks if handles needle	–2
• Dressing suggested	1
• Removal of sutures in 7 days	1
Warns about signs of infection	1
Advises when to return if worried	1
Advises to cover wound for work	1
Invites questions	1
Demonstrates systematic, organized approach	2
Global score from examiner	5
Global score from actor	5
Total	**35**

Question 22 Shortness of breath 1

Instructions for candidate
This patient has attended the ED because he is feeling out of breath. He is stable, looks well, but is slightly breathless. Please take a history, and explain to the patient what you think is going on.

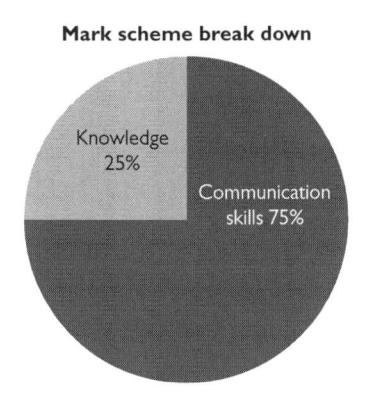

Mark scheme break down

- Knowledge 25%
- Communication skills 75%

Instructions for actor
You are a middle-aged person who has been on renal dialysis for the last 8 years. You went into renal failure because you have polycystic renal disease and you are waiting for a kidney transplant. You dialyse three times a week and have been very stable. You are due to dialyse tomorrow morning.

In the last few months, you have become increasingly frustrated with having dialysis, and are resentful that you haven't been offered a kidney transplant yet. You have become more relaxed about fluid balance, drinking more than you should, prior to dialysis. This week, you have had friends to stay, and have had a few dinner parties, where you have had more glasses of wine than your fluid balance allows. You have been gradually getting more out of breath over the last 48 hours.

You have never had any problems with your breathing before. You don't smoke or have any other medical problems. You haven't had any chest pain.

Instructions for examiner
Observation only.

Equipment required
None

Curriculum mapping
Sections of the CEM (2010) curriculum relevant to this question include the following.

Common competencies

CC1 History taking
CC3 Therapeutics and safe prescribing
CC4 Time management and decision-making
CC5 Decision-making and clinical reasoning
CC6 Patient as the central focus of care
CC12 Relationship with patients and communication

ACCS Acute presentations CT1&2
CAP6 Breathlessness

Mark scheme

Introduces self	1
Checks patient is comfortable	1
Ensures patient is well enough to continue giving history (rather than requiring any acute management)	1
Obtains history of presenting complaint:	
• Nature of dyspnoea	1
• Elicits reasons for attendance	1
• Duration	1
• Severity	1
• Previous episodes	1
Elicits differential negatives	
• Cough	1
• Chest pain	1
• Haemoptysis	1
• Other systemic features, e.g. fever	1
Obtains past medical history	1
Establishes renal history	1
Establishes dialysis history:	
• Pattern and frequency	1
• Last session	1
• Next session	1
Establishes fluid balance:	
• Normal urine output	1
• Normal weight	1
Elicits reasons for poor fluid balance	1
Demonstrates poor compliance with fluid restrictions	1
Explores patient's understanding of fluid balance	1
Asks about drug history	1
Asks about social history	1
Asks about allergies	1
Asks about family history	1
Explains differential diagnosis	1
Carries out differential diagnosis to include pulmonary oedema	1
Explains need to examine and investigate (urine and electrolytes (U&E), CXR, ECG)	1
Confirms need to contact patient's normal renal team	1
Invites questions	1
Global score from examiner	5
Global score from actor	5
Total	**41**

Question 23 Respiratory system examination

Instructions for candidate
This patient has attended the ED with a cough and feeling mildly unwell. Please examine this patient's respiratory system, and then explain your findings and management plan to the patient.

Mark scheme break down

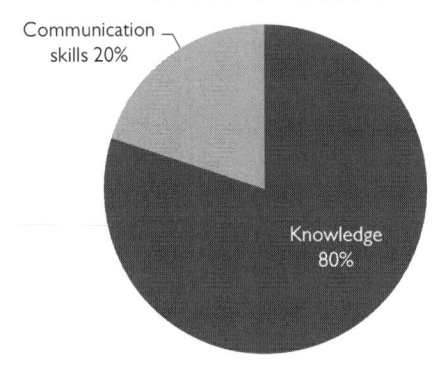

- Communication skills 20%
- Knowledge 80%

Instructions for actor
The candidate will examine you. You are comfortable and not out of breath. After examining you, the candidate should tell you that everything seems normal. They should then tell you what they want to do next. If the candidate does not tell you anything, you should ask them the following questions:

'What do you think is wrong with me?'
'Do I need any tests?'
'What treatment are you going to give me?'
'Can I go home now?'

Instructions for examiner
Observation only.

Equipment required
None

Curriculum mapping
Sections of the CEM (2010) curriculum relevant to this question include the following.

Common competencies

CC2 Clinical examination
CC6 Patient as the central focus of care
CC10 Infection control
CC12 Relationship with patients and communication

ACCS Acute presentations CT1&2

CAP6 Breathlessness
CAP9 Cough
CAP23 Pain management

Question 23 Respiratory system examination

Mark scheme

Introduces self	1
Washes hands	1
Checks patient is comfortable	1
Carries out inspection—general, e.g. comfortable, using oxygen, able to complete sentences comfortably	1
Offers chaperone	1
Adequately exposes chest and abdomen	1
Inspects hands—clubbing, nicotine staining	2
Assesses adequate timing of pulse rate	1
Assesses adequate timing of respiratory rate (RR)	1
Inspects face—checks for cyanosis/anaemia	1
Inspects and palpates neck—checks for enlarged lymph nodes in cervical, supraclavicular, and infraclavicular regions, trachea central, JVP	1
Inspects chest for scars, asymmetrical movements, etc.	1
Examines front, back, and sides of patient	1
Palpates for symmetrical chest expansion	1
Carries out percussion of chest	1
Carries out auscultation of chest in apex, axilla, upper/mid/lower zones	1
Allows patient to get dressed afterwards	1
Explains findings (normal examination) to patient	1
Invites questions	1
Gives advice about further management, e.g. simple analgesics, cough syrup, fluids, probably viral illness, return if worried	2
Demonstrates systematic, organized approach	2
Global score from examiner	5
Global score from actor	5
Total	**34**

Question 24 Child protection

Instructions for candidate

Please take a focused history from the mother of a child (Emma) who has been brought in with a burned hand. The notes written by the triage nurse indicate that the injury happened 2 days ago. When you have taken a history, please examine the child's hand (only) and then explain to the mother what you would like to do next.

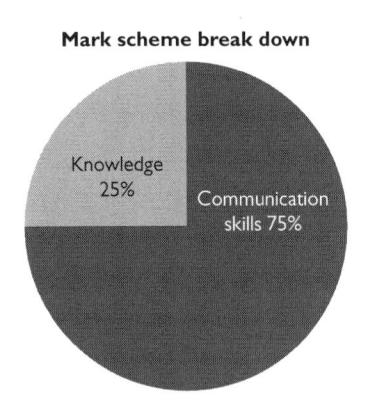

Mark scheme break down

- Knowledge 25%
- Communication skills 75%

Instructions for actor

You are the mother of this 1-year-old child, Emma, who burned her hand 2 days ago. You don't know how it happened because Emma was left with a friend and her boyfriend, and you were not there at the time because you were out with a new boyfriend. You have not asked the friend how the burn happened because you don't want to upset her and risk losing your only babysitter. You are worried that this story will sound bad to the doctors and nurses, so you make up a story about how the burn happened.

You tell them that you were in the kitchen at home, doing the ironing, with Emma playing on the kitchen floor. The phone rang and you went into the hallway to answer it. It was a friend phoning for a chat, but you were only out of the room for a few seconds. When you came back in, Emma was sitting with the iron on the floor, crying, and you noticed the burn on her hand. You washed it under cold water and gave her some paracetamol, and did not come to hospital because you thought it would be fine. You have only come in today because it hasn't healed yet.

The real story, is that you haven't had time to come to hospital because you have been going out with your new boyfriend so much. You worry that the doctors will take the child away from you if you tell them the truth, so you make up answers to any questions they ask, to make your story more plausible.

The child is normally fit and well, and has had all her vaccinations. You had Emma when you were 18 years old, and you no longer have any contact with her father. You have recently moved to the area and you live in a flat alone and have no family nearby. You have made a couple of friends at the local pub who babysit when you want to go out. You used to have regular contact with the health visitor until you moved house, but, since moving, you haven't had a chance to register with a GP, so haven't been put in touch with the health visitor. You are unemployed and find it difficult to find money to live off. You and Emma have never had any contact with social services. You had an uneventful pregnancy, and Emma was born at full term by forceps delivery. There were no problems when she was a newborn baby, and you have been told that she is gaining weight and developing normally.

Question 24 Child protection

You get very defensive if the candidate is suspicious of Emma's injury. You ask the candidate: 'Are you going to take her off me?' If the candidate tries to explain that they are going to refer you to see a health visitor, or social worker, you ask them: 'Are you accusing me of child abuse?' If the candidate wants you both to stay in hospital, you are initially very reluctant but allow yourself to be persuaded. No matter how much you are questioned, you do not reveal the true story about Emma's burn.

Instructions for examiner

Allow the candidate to take a history. After 5 minutes, if they have not examined Emma's hand, you should interrupt and suggest that they are more than half way through and they should examine the child, and then explain the management to Emma's mother.

When the candidate examines Emma's hand, explain that there is a circular, well-circumscribed burn, measuring about 1 cm, in the centre of the baby's palm (i.e. not consistent with the story given).

Equipment required

Infant manikin to sit on actor's lap, with simulated burn on palm of hand

Curriculum mapping

Sections of the CEM (2010) curriculum relevant to this question include the following.

Common competencies

CC1 History taking
CC2 Clinical examination
CC4 Time management and decision-making
CC5 Decision-making and clinical reasoning
CC6 Patient as the central focus of care
CC7 Prioritization of patient safety in clinical practice
CC12 Relationship with patients and communication

Paediatric acute presentations (PAPs)

PAP6 Concerning presentations

Guidelines available

http://www.collemergencymed.ac.uk/shop-floor/clinical%20guidelines/ clinical%20guidelines/default.asp, then follow **Safeguarding Children**

Mark scheme

Introduces self	1
Asks child's name and checks mother's relationship	1
Uses open questions to establish history	1
Establishes details of story	2
Establishes reason for delay in presentation	2
Asks about Emma's medical history, including vaccinations	2
Asks about pregnancy, birth, perinatal problems, Emma's development and weight gain	2
Asks about previous contact with health visitor, social services, and GP	1
Briefly examines child's hand	1

Continued

Continued

Indicates to examiner that a complete examination of child is necessary (examiner will indicate that this examination is normal)	1
Ensures adequate management of burn, e.g. cleaning, analgesia, dressing +/− specialist review	1
States to parents that they are concerned about type of injury and delay in presentation	1
Advises referral to child protection team in a sensitive but firm way	2
Asks that they do not leave hospital until seen	1
Gives thorough explanation to mother	2
Invites questions	1
Global score from examiner	5
Global score from actor	5
Total	**32**

Question 25 Breaking bad news 2

Instructions for candidate

You are the registrar on duty overnight when a 19-year-old student (Jane Smith) is brought in by ambulance, having been knocked off her moped on her way to university. She was unconscious at the scene and had several severe injuries. About 10 minutes after arriving in the department, she had a cardiac arrest. Despite full resuscitation attempts from you and your team, after an hour, with no return of spontaneous circulation, you stopped resuscitation and she was pronounced dead. During resuscitation, she was intubated and ventilated, had bilateral chest drains inserted, several units of blood transfused, and a pelvic sling applied.

The girl's mother has just arrived in the department and does not know what has happened. The ED reception staff have put the girl's mother in the relatives room. Explain to the girl's mother that her daughter has died.

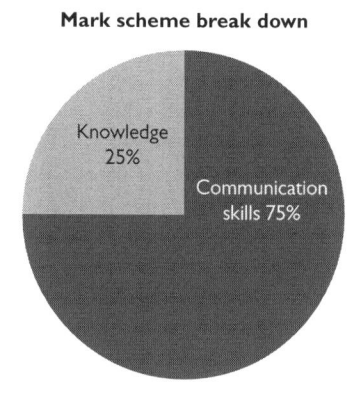

Mark scheme break down

- Knowledge 25%
- Communication skills 75%

Instructions for actor

You are Jane Smith's mother. You had a phone call on your mobile phone about 2 hours ago from an 'ambulance man' who told you Jane had come off her moped and had been injured. They told you she was being taken to the nearest hospital and advised you to go straight there. Your husband, Jane's father, is away in Singapore on a business trip. Jane is an only child.

You have no idea that Jane has been seriously injured. You are shocked and disbelieving when you are told she is dead. You want to know why the doctor has 'given up' on her. You are devastated that your only child is dead. When you are offered the chance to see Jane, you find the idea very upsetting and refuse.

You know that Jane was not on the organ donor register, and would not like to discuss this further. If the candidate suggests phoning someone, you explain that your husband is away. You eventually are persuaded to phone your sister, who lives nearby.

Instructions for examiner

Observation only.

If the candidate asks for another member of staff for assistance, e.g. a nurse to accompany them, state that there is no-one available at the present but that one will be ready in 10 minutes time.

Equipment required

None

Curriculum mapping

Sections of the CEM (2010) curriculum relevant to this question include the following.

Common competencies

CC5 Decision-making and clinical reasoning
CC6 Patient as the central focus of care
CC7 Prioritization of patient safety in clinical practice
CC12 Relationship with patients and communication
CC13 Breaking bad news

ACCS Major presentations CT1&2

CMP3 Major trauma

Mark scheme

Chooses suitable location (e.g. relatives room, not resus)	1
Ensures bleep/mobile switched off	1
Lets departmental staff know location	1
Asks for a nurse to accompany them	1
Introduces self	1
Checks correct identity	1
Establishes what is already known	1
Explains diagnosis clearly and without delay	2
Uses the words 'died' or 'dead'	1
Asks about other relatives	1
Invites questions/allows suitable pauses for questions	1
Offers pastoral support	1
Introduces idea of organ donation	1
Offers chance to see body	1
Offers nurse to sit with afterwards	1
Answers questions adequately and sensitively	2
Appropriately uses silence	1
Global score from examiner	5
Global score from actor	5
Total	**29**

Question 26 Asthma

Instructions for candidate
A 7-year-old boy, James, is brought to hospital by his parents after becoming wheezy overnight. He is known to have asthma and it is usually quite well controlled on a salbutamol inhaler used as required. However, in the last couple of weeks he has been using his inhaler more often than normal.

He became very wheezy at school today and the school nurse called an ambulance. He was given a salbutamol nebulizer and now feels much better. He has been observed in the ED for 2 hours and is ready to be discharged. His peak flow is within normal range for him and he has no features of severe asthma. Please give James and his parents the necessary information prior to being discharged.

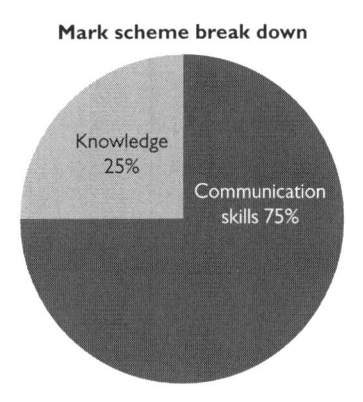

Mark scheme break down

- Knowledge 25%
- Communication skills 75%

Instructions for actor 1 (child)
You have had an asthma attack for the first time and been brought into hospital by ambulance from school. You felt a bit wheezy at school and asked your teacher for your inhaler. The teacher took you to see the nurse, who called for an ambulance. You didn't feel that bad, and it was very exciting to get a ride in an ambulance. You're bored of waiting in hospital and want to go home. You don't feel wheezy anymore and can almost get your normal score on your peak flow monitor. You have been on a blue inhaler since you were little, but only seem to get wheezy when you have a cold or have hay fever (runny nose and itchy eyes). You have never had any other type of inhaler. You don't use a volumatic; you just squirt the inhaler into your mouth at the same time as taking a deep breath. If the doctor shows you how to use the volumatic, you get the hang of it quickly.

Instructions for actor 2 (parent)
You have never seen a volumatic before so you need to be instructed how to use it. You have not seen an asthma nurse before, and haven't taken James to the GP for a couple of years because he hardly ever seems to need his inhaler. You're not sure exactly what to do when James gets wheezy—he has looked after his own inhalers for the last year or so. The inhaler you have at the moment is running out because he has been using it so much in the last couple of days.

Instructions for examiner
Observation only. This patient's presentation does not require oral steroid but the candidate should be allowed to consider this option, as local practice varies.

Equipment required
Standard salbutamol metered dose inhaler
Standard size volumatic

Self-Assessment for the MCEM Part C

Curriculum mapping

Sections of the CEM (2010) curriculum relevant to this question include the following.

Common competencies

CC1 History taking
CC2 Clinical examination
CC3 Therapeutics and safe prescribing
CC4 Time management and decision-making
CC5 Decision-making and clinical reasoning
CC6 Patient as the central focus of care
CC7 Prioritization of patient safety in clinical practice
CC11 Management of long-term conditions and promoting patient self-care
CC12 Relationship with patients and communication
CC16 Health promotion and public health

Paediatric acute presentations (PAPs)

PAP5 Breathing difficulties—recognize the critically ill and those who will need intubation and ventilation

Guidelines available

http://www.brit-thoracic.org.uk/guidelines/asthma-guidelines.aspx

Mark scheme

Introduces self	1
Checks identity of James and/or parent	1
Explains plan is to discharge home	1
Explains what to do in emergency	2
Explains patient needs 'preventer' inhaler in addition	1
Explains volumatic	1
Explains need to use salbutamol **before** preventer	1
Checks technique adequately:	
• Asks patient to demonstrate their inhaler use	1
• Describes adequate technique	1
• Demonstrates technique	1
• Checks patient is able to reproduce technique	1
Checks if needs new salbutamol inhaler/checks current inhaler full and in date	1
Provides and/or explains written asthma plan	1
Advises follow-up (GP or asthma nurse)	1
Safety netting—gives guidance about when to represent	1
Explains emergency management of asthma	3
Invites questions	1
Global score from examiner	5
Global score from actors	5
Total	**30**

Question 27 Knee examination

Instructions for candidate
This young football player has hurt his knee an hour ago during a tackle. He can weight bear but it is painful. Please examine his knee and explain to the patient what your management will involve.

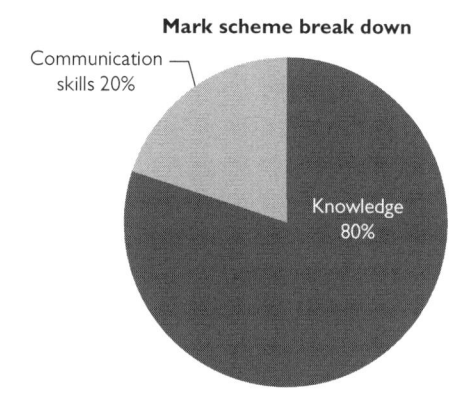

Mark scheme break down
- Communication skills 20%
- Knowledge 80%

Instructions for actor
You are a keen amateur footballer and also work as a self-employed carpet fitter. You were in football training when you were tackled badly and twisted your knee. You can walk on it but it is very painful. You have no medical problems and take no medications.

If the candidate asks you to walk, you can, but tell them it hurts your knee. If they ask you to move the knee, you are able, but it hurts to straighten your leg fully. If they touch your knee, the only area that is sore is the anterior joint line. The other tests that they do to your knee are not painful.

Instructions for examiner
Allow the candidate to examine the knee and explain their management to the patient. If the candidate gets to the last minute of the station and has not started to explain anything to the patient, prompt them that they have a minute left, so they should move on to explaining their management.

Equipment required
None

Curriculum mapping
Sections of the CEM (2010) curriculum relevant to this question include the following.

Common competencies
CC2 Clinical examination
CC3 Therapeutics and safe prescribing
CC4 Time management and decision-making
CC5 Decision-making and clinical reasoning
CC6 Patient as the central focus of care
CC11 Management of long-term conditions and promoting patient self-care
CC12 Relationship with patients and communication

ACCS Acute presentations CT1&2

CAP23 Pain management
CAP33 Traumatic limb and joint injuries

Mark scheme

Introduces self	1
Offers chaperone	1
Washes hands	1
Ensures patient comfortable—check analgesia given or required	1
Assesses gait/weight bearing (can be done at end of examination)	1
Exposes both knees from thigh to calf	1
Compares left with right throughout	1
Observes:	
• Varus/valgus deformity	1
• Swelling	1
• Muscle wasting	1
• Scars/signs of previous injury/surgery	1
• Trauma/bruising	1
Comments on relevant negatives	1
Palpates and checks for:	
• Temperature difference	1
• Effusion/patella tap	1
• Joint lines including proximal fibula, distal femur, tibial tuberosity, popliteal fossa	1
Carries out thorough assessment of movements:	
• Straight leg raise	1
• Active flexion/extension	1
• Passive flexion/extension	1
Carries out special tests:	
• Anterior and posterior cruciate ligaments	1
• Medial collateral ligament and lateral collateral ligament stress test	1
• McMurray's test	1
• Patella apprehension test	1
Carries out neurovascular examination	2
Offers to examine hip and ankle joint	1
Demonstrates systematic, organized approach	2
Summarizes findings	3
Suggests diagnosis and ongoing management plan	2
Specifically addresses work- and sports-related issues, e.g. return to work and sport	1
Global score from examiner	5
Global score from actor	5
Total	**44**

Question 28 Chest pain 2

Instructions for candidate

Take a history from this patient who has attended the ED with chest pain. Clinical examination is normal and the patient is stable. His ECG is normal and the pain is now settled. His initial troponin, taken an hour after the onset of pain, has come back within normal limits. After taking a history, explain to him what your management plan is.

Mark scheme break down

- Knowledge 25%
- Communication skills 75%

Instructions for actor

You are a 40-year-old builder who has had a 20-minute episode of central chest pain, which radiated down both arms. The pain came on after you had been loading some supplies onto your lorry earlier today. Your workmates said you looked sweaty and they called an ambulance. When the paramedics arrived, they gave you some spray under your tongue and the pain went away. You now feel fine. The pain lasted about 20 minutes in total.

You have had this pain several times before but have never told anyone about it. It usually comes on after doing activity, such as loading the lorry, gardening, or playing football with your sons. Usually it goes away after about 20 minutes, if you rest.

You deny having previous medical problems, but you have been told you have high BP by your GP, though you don't take any medication for it because you don't like going to the doctors. You have no family history. Your older brother has had a heart attack in his 40s. You have no other medical problems and don't smoke. You have a very active job, and play football with your sons in the garden a few times a week. You are keen to go home but go along with whatever the doctor advises.

Instructions for examiner

Observation only.

Equipment required

Normal ECG

Curriculum mapping

Sections of the CEM (2010) curriculum relevant to this question include the following.

Common competencies

CC1 History taking
CC3 Therapeutics and safe prescribing

CC4 Time management and decision-making
CC5 Decision-making and clinical reasoning
CC6 Patient as the central focus of care
CC7 Prioritization of patient safety in clinical practice
CC12 Relationship with patients and communication

ACCS Acute presentations CT1&2

CAP7 Chest pain
CAP23 Pain management

Mark scheme

Introduces self	1
Asks characteristics of pain	3
Checks associated features	2
Ascertains that pain relieved by glyceryl trinitrate (GTN) spray	1
Asks precipitant of pain	1
Asks about previous episodes of pain	1
Asks about cardiac risk factors	3
Asks about exercise	1
Asks about family history	1
Asks about past medical history	1
Explains patient needs additional investigation, including delayed cardiac enzymes (e.g. troponin at 6 hours, depending on local protocols)	1
Explains that diagnosis at this stage includes cardiac problems	1
Explains management options:	
• If delayed cardiac enzymes normal—will be discharged home, but needs follow-up in chest pain clinic due to risk factors	2
• If delayed cardiac enzymes abnormal—will be admitted to hospital under cardiology team for further investigation, including angiogram, and treatment	2
Invites questions	1
Global score from examiner	5
Global score from actor	5
Total	**32**

Question 29 Headache

Instructions for candidate

Take a history from this patient who has attended the ED with a headache, and then explain your management plan.

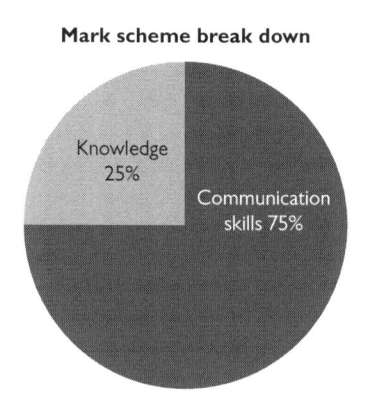

Mark scheme break down

- Knowledge 25%
- Communication skills 75%

Instructions for actor

You are a 52-year-old woman who has attended the ED with a severe headache. You have never had a headache like this before. It came on suddenly while you were driving to visit your daughter's house nearby. It made you feel sick and dizzy, and you had to stop the car in the road straight away. You did not lose consciousness/pass out but you felt vey unwell. A passerby called an ambulance. When it arrived, you vomited several times and you still feel very nauseous.

The pain was severe (10 out of 10) and is all over your head, radiating into your neck. You were given some painkillers and antisickness through a drip by the ambulance crew, and you feel a bit more comfortable. You didn't have any other symptoms at the same time as the pain. Specifically, no facial or limb weakness, your vision was unchanged, and your speech was normal throughout.

You have no previous medical problems and don't smoke or take any medications. You are a head teacher and you cycle 4 miles to work every day. You are divorced from your husband and have three grown-up children who live nearby. You have never suffered from migraines. Your father had a stroke before he died, age 78. Your mother is still alive at the age of 80 and has high BP only. You are happy to go along with whatever the doctor recommends.

Instructions for examiner

Observation only.

Equipment required

None

Curriculum mapping

Sections of the CEM (2010) curriculum relevant to this question include the following.

Common competencies

CC1 History taking
CC4 Time management and decision-making
CC5 Decision-making and clinical reasoning

CC6 Patient as the central focus of care
CC12 Relationship with patients and communication

ACCS Acute presentations CT1&2
CAP17 Headache
CAP23 Pain management

Guidelines available

http://www.collemergencymed.ac.uk/shop-floor/clinical%20guidelines/clinical%20guidelines/default.asp, then follow **Lone Acute Severe Headache**

Mark scheme

Introduces self	1
Ensures patient is comfortable and offers analgesia	1
Assesses nature of pain:	
• Character	1
• Duration	1
• Precipitating factors	1
• Relieving factors	1
Looks for associated features:	
• Vomiting	1
• Limb or facial weakness	1
• Slurred speech	1
• Visual disturbance	1
• 'Auras'	1
Asks about previous headaches, e.g. migraine frequency and triggers	1
Obtains past medical history and drug history	1
Asks about recent medication changes	1
Asks about anticoagulants	1
Asks about social history	1
Asks about family history	1
Explains possible diagnosis:	
• Common: tensions headaches, migraine, cluster headaches	1
• Uncommon but important: subarachnoid haemorrhage	1
Explains management:	
• Clinical examination including full neurological examination	1
• CT head scan	1
• Admit to ward/observation unit and do lumbar puncture (LP) at 12 hours post onset of headache	2
Global score from examiner	5
Global score from actor	5
Total	**32**

Question 30 Ear pain

Instructions for candidate
Please take a history from the mother of this toddler who has been brought to the ED because of ear pain, and explain to the child's mother what your management will be.

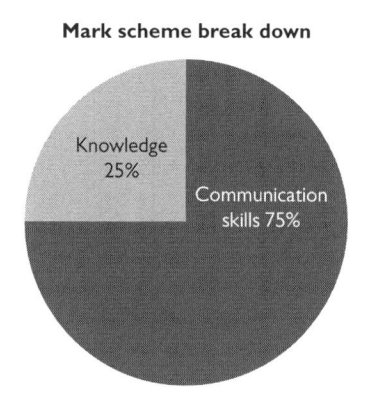

Mark scheme break down

- Knowledge 25%
- Communication skills 75%

Instructions for actor
You are the mother of a 20-month-old child, Sam, who has been miserable for the last 24 hours. You think he has an ear infection because he had a snotty nose last week, and in the last 2 days he has been pulling his ears and crying more than normal. He is eating and drinking and has had some mild fevers. He has not had any diarrhoea or vomiting and has been well enough to go to nursery throughout the illness. He sometimes wakes up during the night and seems difficult to settle, which is unusual for him, and he seems more tired than normal. He has not had any other symptoms. You have brought him in to the ED in the hope that you might get some antibiotics so that Sam can get back to normal. You have been giving him paracetamol every now and again during this illness, but it doesn't seem to make much difference.

Sam is normally well, has not been in hospital before, and takes no medications. He gets mild eczema from time to time that you put cream on, which usually settles it down. He has an older sister, 4-year-old Ellie, who has also had a runny nose and sore throat in the last week or so. He has had several colds before, which you think he catches from the other children at nursery. He has had all of his vaccinations, and had an uneventful birth and perinatal period, after a normal pregnancy.

You are an intensive care nurse who works full time. Sam goes to nursery 3 days a week, your mother looks after him on one day, and you look after him on the other days between your shifts. After taking a history, the candidate should advise you about what to do with Sam. If the candidate does not specifically mention antibiotics, then ask them 'Doesn't he need some antibiotics to clear this up once and for all?'

Instructions for examiner
Observation only.

Equipment required
None

Curriculum mapping
Sections of the CEM (2010) curriculum relevant to this question include the following.

Common competencies

CC1 History taking
CC3 Therapeutics and safe prescribing
CC4 Time management and decision-making
CC5 Decision-making and clinical reasoning
CC6 Patient as the central focus of care
CC11 Management of long-term conditions and promoting patient self-care
CC12 Relationship with patients and communication

Paediatric acute presentations (PAPs)

PAP8 ENT
PAP9 Fever in all age groups
PAP15 Pain in children

Guidelines available

http://www.collemergencymed.ac.uk/shop-floor/clinical%20guidelines/clinical%20guidelines/default.asp, then follow **Pain in Children**

http://publications.nice.org.uk/cg69

Mark scheme

Introduces self	1
Checks identity	1
Uses open questions to establish history	3
Establishes characteristics of ear pain and coryzal symptoms	2
Asks about fever	1
Asks about eating and drinking/wet nappies	1
Asks about other symptoms, e.g. diarrhoea and vomiting, rash	2
Asks about social history	1
Asks about immunizations	1
Asks about past medical problems/medications/allergies	2
Asks about birth/perinatal history	1
Asks about developmental milestones, specifically speech and language	1
Asks about previous hearing tests	1
Discusses management:	
• Natural history of illness (self-limiting illness lasting 4–5 days)	2
• Plan to examine child	1
• No need for antibiotics (makes little difference to symptoms and can cause diarrhoea)	2
• Advice about regular analgesia	1
Safety netting—offers advice about seeking medical attention if deteriorates and follow-up with GP	1
Global score from examiner	5
Global score from actor	5
Total	**35**

Question 31 Diarrhoea and vomiting

Instructions for candidate
Please take a history from the parent of this 4-year-old child, Jack, who has been brought to the ED because he has had diarrhoea and vomiting.

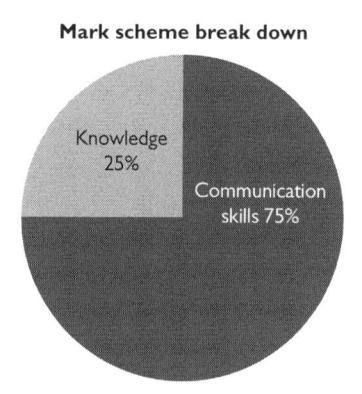

Mark scheme break down

- Knowledge 25%
- Communication skills 75%

Instructions for actor
You are the parent of a 4-year-old child, Jack, who has had diarrhoea and vomiting for the last 2 days. You have brought Jack to hospital because he has got worse today and is now vomiting every time you give him any fluid, and you are worried he will get dehydrated.

There is a vomiting bug going around his class, and lots of his friends had the same thing a few days ago. It started 2 days ago, when Jack said he wasn't hungry and then vomited once before he went to bed. Overnight he vomited twice but seemed better the next morning. But that afternoon, the vomiting started again, this time with diarrhoea. Yesterday Jack vomited every 2 hours or so and had four episodes of loose watery stool. Today he vomits every time you give him anything to drink, but has not had any diarrhoea for several hours. You think he has been a bit hot and bothered but hasn't had any high fevers.

You are a bit worried about him today because he hasn't had a wee all day and seems completely exhausted. He has been lying in his bed and doesn't even want to come downstairs and lie on the sofa to watch television. He has been sleeping more than usual, but when you go in to his bedroom, he wakes up and asks you for a drink. He has not been unconscious or unresponsive at any time. He seems weak but has not been limp or floppy. He feels nice and warm all over, but you think he looks a bit pale.

Jack is normally a very healthy child. He has mild asthma for which he takes a blue inhaler when he gets wheezy, which is only when he has a cold. He had eczema as a baby and toddler but seems to have grown out of it now. He has an older sister, Holly, who is 7 years old. She has also been unwell with this bug, but only had a couple of episodes of vomiting and mild diarrhoea. She is now better and back at school.

Jack was born by elective caesarean section at 39 weeks because he was a breech baby. Your pregnancy was uneventful and there were no problems when he was a newborn baby. He has had all of his immunizations. Jack lives with you, his sister, and father. You work part time as a cleaner and look after the children. Both children are in school nearby.

Instructions for examiner
Observation only.

Equipment required
None

Curriculum mapping
Sections of the CEM (2010) curriculum relevant to this question include the following.

Common competencies
CC1 History taking
CC4 Time management and decision-making
CC6 Patient as the central focus of care
CC12 Relationship with patients and communication

Paediatric acute presentations (PAPs)
PAP1 Abdominal pain
PAP7 Dehydration secondary to diarrhoea and vomiting
PAP9 Fever in all age groups

Guideline
http://publications.nice.org.uk/cg84

Mark scheme

Introduces self	1
Checks identity	1
Uses open questions to establish history	1
Asks about:	
• Contacts	1
• Foreign travel	1
Asks about characteristics of symptoms:	
• Number of vomits in 24 hours	1
• Number of episodes of diarrhoea in last 24 hours	1
Asks about fever	1
Asks about eating and drinking, passing urine	2
Asks about other symptoms to exclude alternative significant diagnoses:	
• Rash	1
• Urinary symptoms	1
• SOB	1
• Blood/mucus in stool	1
• Bilious green vomiting	1
Asks about social history	1
Asks about immunizations	1
Asks about past medical problems/medications/allergies	1
Obtains birth/perinatal history	1

Continued

Question 31 Diarrhoea and vomiting

Continued

Discusses management:	
• Plans to examine child	1
• Looks for markers of dehydration and mentions 'red flags'	1
• Discusses no antibiotics	1
• Advises about regular paracetamol	1
• Discourages fruit juice/carbonated drinks	1
• Offers rehydration salt solution and advises volume (5 ml/kg after each large watery stool)	1
Safety netting—offers advice about medical help/GP follow-up	1
Offers hygiene advice, e.g. hand washing	1
Offers child care advice—advises no contact for 48 hours after symptoms resolve	1
Global score from examiner	5
Global score from actor	5
Total	**39**

Question 32 Femoral line

Instructions for candidate
This 32-year-old IV drug user, John, has presented to the ED with a 2-day history of severe abdominal pain and vomiting. John tells you he is an alcoholic and has had pancreatitis in the past. He looks pale and sweaty, with a BP of 90/60 and HR of 120. He has no accessible peripheral veins, and needs IV fluids. Please insert a femoral central venous access line into the model provided. The actor will play the role of John, but the central line should be inserted into the model.

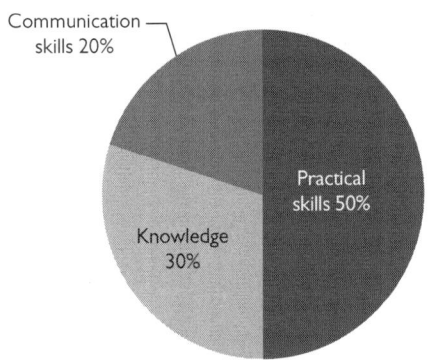

Mark scheme break down
- Communication skills 20%
- Practical skills 50%
- Knowledge 30%

Instructions for actor
You have been brought to hospital by ambulance with severe abdominal pain and vomiting. You have had pancreatitis in the past and it feels like the same thing. Your veins have disappeared from injecting drugs for several years. At present, you inject into your neck veins. On the last few times you were in hospital, you have had to have central lines. You know what is involved and go along with what the candidate advises.

Equipment required
Model for femoral line access
Cleaning solution
Sterile gloves, gown, and mask
Gauze swabs
Ultrasound machine
Local anaesthetic
Sterile saline
Selection of needles and syringes
Introducers
Guide wire
Scalpel
Central venous catheter
Sutures
Dressings

Instructions for examiner
Ensure that the candidate is aware they should carry out the procedure on the model, not the actor. When the candidate indicates that they would like to wash their hands and use personal protective

Question 32 Femoral line

equipment, tell them to proceed without actually doing so, to save time. Do not award a mark for this if the candidate does not mention it.

Curriculum mapping
Sections of the CEM (2010) curriculum relevant to this question include the following.

Common competencies
CC2 Clinical examination
CC3 Therapeutics and safe prescribing
CC4 Time management and decision-making
CC6 Patient as the central focus of care
CC7 Prioritization of patient safety in clinical practice
CC8 Team work and patient safety
CC10 Infection control
CC12 Relationship with patients and communication
CC18 Valid consent

ACCS Major presentations CT1&2
CMP5 Shocked patient

ACCS Acute presentations CT1&2
CAP1 Abdominal pain including loin pain
CAP23 Pain management
CAP36 Vomiting and nausea

Mark scheme

Introduces self	1
Checks identity	1
Explains procedure	2
Obtains verbal consent, assent	1
Gathers correct equipment	2
Ensures correct patient position	1
Uses sterile technique (washes hands, uses gown, gloves, and mask)	1
Flushes line with saline	1
Uses ultrasound to identify anatomy or in real time	1
Local anaesthetic—uses correct dose depending on agent selected	1
Identifies femoral vein with needle and syringe	1
Introduce guide wire	1
Opens track with dilators and scalpel to skin	1
Positions catheter	1
Aspirates and flushes catheter ports	1
Secures catheter with sutures	1
Applies dressing	1
Allows patient to sit up, reassures, offers painkillers	1

Continued

Self-Assessment for the MCEM Part C

Continued

Thanks patient	1
Clears sharps	2
Global score from examiner	5
Global score from actor	5
Total	**34**

Question 33 Neck injury 1

Instructions for candidate

This 80-year-old man fell over yesterday in the street whilst he was doing his shopping. He tripped on a step and fell forwards. He was unable to put his hands out to save himself and banged his chin on the pavement. At the time, his neck hurt a bit, but he picked himself up and slowly made his way home. He has come to the ED today because his arms feel weak.

He is in a cubicle where he is immobilized in a semirigid collar, sand bags, and tape. He has already been log-rolled, which was normal. Please examine this patient and explain to him what your management will be.

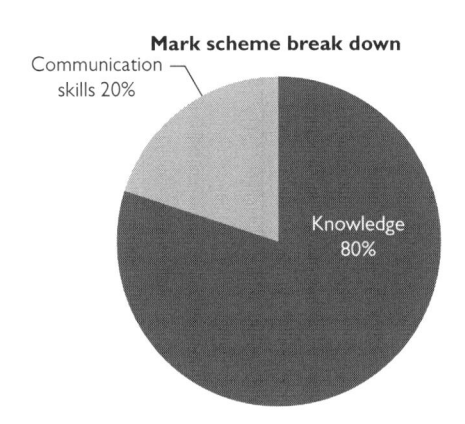

Mark scheme break down
- Communication skills 20%
- Knowledge 80%

Instructions for actor

You are immobilized in a semirigid collar, sand bags, and tape. You are an elderly man who fell over yesterday while you were doing your shopping. You were carrying two bags so you couldn't put your arms out, and banged your chin badly on the pavement when you fell. You have a bruised face and a sore neck. You managed to make your way slowly home yesterday, but this morning you have woken up with weak arms and altered sensation in your arms.

When the candidate examines the strength of your upper limbs, you find you are weak throughout the arms, and although you try to follow their commands, you cannot lift your arms off the bed. When the candidate tests the sensation in your arms, you can feel them touching you but it feels 'a bit numb' all over. The rest of your body, including your legs and face, are completely normal.

Instructions for examiner

The patient has central cord syndrome. Observation only. You may ask the candidate what they think the most likely diagnosis is.

Equipment required

Examination trolley
Selection of cervical collars
'Sand bags'
Tape

Curriculum mapping

Sections of the CEM (2010) curriculum relevant to this question include the following.

Self-Assessment for the MCEM Part C

Common competencies

CC1 History taking
CC2 Clinical examination
CC4 Time management and decision-making
CC5 Decision-making and clinical reasoning
CC12 Relationship with patients and communication

ACCS Acute presentations CT1&2

CAP18 Head injury
CAP21 Neck pain
CAP23 Pain management
CAP37 Weakness and paralysis

Mark scheme

Introduces self	1
Offers chaperone	1
Examines upper limb:	
• Inspection	1
• Tone	1
• Power	1
• Reflexes	1
• Sensation	1
• Coordination	1
Examines lower limb:	
• Inspection	1
• Tone	1
• Power	1
• Reflexes	1
• Sensation	1
• Coordination	
Explains differential diagnosis—missed fracture, cord compression, central cord syndrome	2
Mentions most likely diagnosis is central cord syndrome (can be directly questioned by examiner)	1
Advises CT scan and/or magnetic resonance imaging (MRI) scan depending on local policy	1
Advises neurosurgical referral	1
Thanks patient	2
Global score from examiner	5
Global score from actor	5
Total	**30**

Question 34 Airway skills

Instructions for candidate

You are in the ED. You have been pre-alerted from the ambulance crew that they are bringing in a 25-year-old man who was found unconscious in the street. He has not responded to a dose of intra-muscular (IM) naloxone and is requiring bag valve mask (BVM) ventilation to support his breathing. They will be arriving in 1 minute. IV access has been secured.

You have a nurse working with you who has no advanced airway training but can pass you any equipment from the airway trolley. Please assess the patient and manage them as necessary.

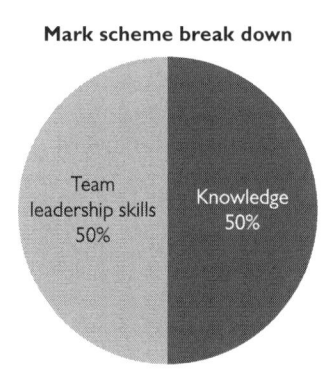

Mark scheme break down

- Team leadership skills 50%
- Knowledge 50%

Instructions for actor

You are a staff nurse who is fairly new to the ED. You know where all the equipment is kept and can hand it to the candidate, but you don't act without being clearly instructed to do so.

Instructions for examiner

The patient is represented by a mannequin. The patient has a standard airway trolley. The patient will arrive after 1 minute, irrespective of what the candidate does. When the candidate requests anaesthetic help, the anaesthetist arrives and encourages the candidate to continue under supervision. If the candidate is unable to intubate the patient, there are marks available for alternative management (see mark scheme). Do not allow the candidate to persist in multiple attempts to intubate.

You can give the following information about the patient to the candidate as they progress through the station:

Airway sounds noisy—not fully cleared with basic airway manoeuvres or adjuncts
Laryngeal mask airway (LMA) leaks
IV access obtained
Observations:
Pulse = 45, BP = 200/110, glucose = 5.2, pupils left = 3 mm, right = 6 mm, GCS = 3

Equipment required

Standard adult resuscitation equipment
Intubating airway manikin

Curriculum mapping

Sections of the CEM (2010) curriculum relevant to this question include the following.

Self-Assessment for the MCEM Part C

Common competencies

CC1 History taking
CC2 Clinical examination
CC3 Therapeutics and safe prescribing
CC4 Time management and decision-making
CC5 Decision-making and clinical reasoning
CC6 Patient as the central focus of care
CC7 Prioritization of patient safety in clinical practice
CC8 Team work and patient safety

ACCS Major presentations CT1&2

CMP6 Unconscious patient

ACCS Acute presentations CT1&2

CAP5 Blackout/collapse
CAP35 Ventilatory support

Mark scheme

Call for senior/anaesthetic assistance	1
Checks:	
• Suction	1
• Laryngoscope ×2—half mark per scope checked	1
• Endotracheal tube (ETT)—cuff check	1
• Appropriate sizes of ETT	1
• Bougie/stylet	1
• Rescue airway device—LMA	1
• End tidal carbon dioxide ($ETCO_2$) monitoring	1
Mentions location of difficult airway equipment	1
Carries out initial assessment of patient airway, breathing, and circulation (ABC)	2
Checks blood glucose	1
Checks oropharyngeal (OP)/nasopharyngeal (NP) airway	1
Uses two-handed technique to optimize airway	1
Inserts LMA (½ mark) but removes as leaking (1½ marks) (if LMA is inserted, examiner should inform candidate that there is a poor seal and ventilation is ineffective)	2
Considers drugs	1
Mentions suitable induction agent, e.g. propofol	1
Mentions muscle relaxant, e.g. suxamethonium	1
Mentions opiates	1
Carries out intubation (maximum of 1 mark only):	1
• Successful first attempt	
• **Or** successful second attempt with manoeuvres to improve view	
• **Or** reverts back to bask-valve mask, LMA, or senior support	

Continued

Question 34 Airway skills

Continued

Institutes post-intubation care:	
Full monitoring	1
Capnography	1
CXR	1
Team leadership skills	2
Global score from examiner	5
Global score from actor	5
Total	**36**

Question 35 Obstetric emergency

Instructions for candidate
You are called to resus to see a 35-year-old lady who is 38 weeks pregnant and has presented with headaches. In triage her BP was noted to be 169/100 mmHg and she has been moved to the resus room for assessment. You have an experienced nurse from the ED with you. Please assess the patient and treat as necessary.

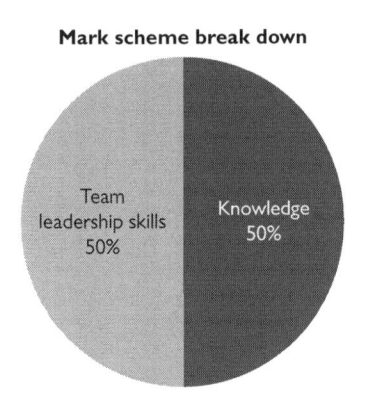

Mark scheme break down

- Team leadership skills 50%
- Knowledge 50%

Instructions for actor 1 (patient)
You are a 35-year-old woman who is 38 weeks pregnant. You are feeling very drowsy because you have just had a seizure. You have had a normal pregnancy so far, with no problems at all, but in the last few days you have started to get bad headaches and notice that your face, arms, and legs are swollen. This is your first pregnancy. You have no medical problems, are not taking any medication, and do not have any allergies.

During the first 2 minutes of the station, you tell the candidate that you are feeling worse. You should start to act drowsy and confused progressively. At a pre-arranged signal from the examiner, at 2 minutes into the station, you should start to simulate having a seizure. The seizure continues until the end of the station.

Instructions for actor 2 (nurse)
You are an experienced staff nurse in the ED. You know where all the equipment is kept and can hand it to the candidate, but you don't act without being clearly instructed to do so.

Instructions for examiner
Allow the candidate to take a history from the candidate. After 2 minutes, signal to the actor that they should start to have a seizure. The seizure continues until the end of the station.

Equipment required
Standard adult resuscitation equipment (see introductory section)
Pillow to mimic third trimester pregnancy
Delivery kit
Neonatal resuscitation kit

Curriculum mapping
Sections of the CEM (2010) curriculum relevant to this question include the following.

Question 35 Obstetric emergency

Common competencies

CC1 History taking
CC2 Clinical examination
CC3 Therapeutics and safe prescribing
CC4 Time management and decision-making
CC5 Decision-making and clinical reasoning
CC6 Patient as the central focus of care
CC7 Prioritization of patient safety in clinical practice
CC8 Team work and patient safety
CC15 Communication with colleagues and cooperation

ACCS Major presentations CT1&2

CMP5 Shocked patient
CMP6 Unconscious patient

ACCS Acute presentations CT1&2

CAP5 Blackout/collapse
CAP15 Fits/seizure
CAP35 Ventilatory support

Guidelines available

http://www.rcog.org.uk/womens-health/clinical-guidance/management-severe-pre-eclampsiaeclampsia-green-top-10a

Mark scheme

Introduces self	1
Obtains focused history of events:	
• Symptoms	1
• Pregnancy	1
• Previous similar problems	1
• Medical history	1
• Drugs	1
Specifically considers markers of pre-eclampsia:	
• Oedema	1
• BP	1
• Proteinuria	1
Offers oxygen	1
Follows A B C D E approach	2
Obtains IV access and sends blood for cross match	1
Asks patient to sit up or left lateral tilt	1
Calls for senior ED help	1
Calls for anaesthetic and obstetric assistance	2
Measures blood glucose	1

Continued

Continued

Offers prompt diagnosis of eclamptic seizure	1
Gives magnesium early (4 g IV)	2
Recognizes need for BP-lowering medication (does not need to know drug names or doses)	1
Considers need for delivery	1
Pre-alerts neonatal team about impending delivery	1
Displays team leadership skills	2
Global score from examiner	5
Global score from actor (nurse)	5
Total	**36**

Question 36 Risk assessment in overdose

Instructions for candidate
Your next patient is a 20-year-old lady who has taken an overdose of paracetamol 3 hours ago. Please take a history from her and explain what you would like to do.

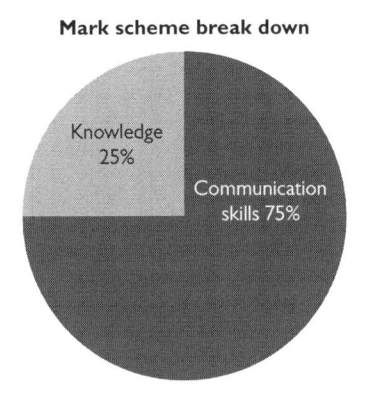

Mark scheme break down

- Knowledge 25%
- Communication skills 75%

Instructions for actor
You have taken 16 paracetamol tablets 3 hours ago because you wanted to die. It is your third overdose in the past 6 months. You are separated from your partner and are a mother of a 3-year-old—who is staying with your ex-partner at weekends (and is there at the moment). You are socially isolated, with no contact with your parents. You can't see the point in going on due to financial problems. You have planned to take the tablets, which you bought from a supermarket last week, for a few days, but you wanted to wait until your daughter was out of the house in case she found your dead body. You only came to hospital because a neighbour came round and found you crying and persuaded you to come in.

You are reluctant to wait in hospital and need to know why a blood test needs to be done and why you might need treatment. If the candidate gives an adequate explanation, you are willing to stay but 'only for the blood test'.

Instructions for examiner
Observation only.

Equipment required
None

Curriculum mapping
Sections of the CEM (2010) curriculum relevant to this question include the following.

Common competencies
CC1 History taking
CC3 Therapeutics and safe prescribing
CC5 Decision-making and clinical reasoning
CC6 Patient as the central focus of care
CC7 Prioritization of patient safety in clinical practice
CC12 Relationship with patients and communication

Self-Assessment for the MCEM Part C

ACCS Acute presentations CT1&2

CAP27 Poisoning
CAP30 Mental health

Guidelines available

http://publications.nice.org.uk/self-harm-cg16
http://secure.collemergencymed.ac.uk/shop-floor/Clinical%20Guidelines/College%20Guidelines/Paracetamol%20Overdose

Mark scheme

Introduces self	1
Establishes tablets taken and timing	1
Ascertains reason for overdose	1
Asks about circumstances—alcohol, reasons, note, etc.	2
Assesses reason for discovery/seeking help	1
Carries out suicide risk assessment using SADPERSONS scale:	10 total for this section
S: Male sex	
A: Older age	
D: Depression	
P: Previous attempt	
E: Ethanol or drug abuse	
R: Rational thinking loss	
S: Social supports lacking	
O: Organized plan	
N: No spouse	
S: Sickness	
Uses results of SADPERSONS score to categorize risk based on the following:	2
0–4 Low	
5–6 Medium	
7–10 High	
Obtains medication history	1
Asks about drug use	1
Asks about past medical history	1
Asks about past psychiatric history	1
Explains need to do paracetamol and salicylate levels at 4 hours post ingestion	1
Explains need to treat if levels abnormal and risks of not treating	1
Advises mental health referral	1
Reviews home situation and discovers dependant minor	1
Explains need to refer to children's services about attendance as carer for child	1
Treats with respect and empathy at all times	1
Offers access to support regarding financial situation, e.g. social services, citizens advice	1
Global score from actor	5
Global score from examiner	5
Total	**39**

Question 37 Eye examination

Instructions for candidate
You are asked to see a 40-year-old man with a painful right eye. Please examine him and discuss your findings and management plan with the examiner.

Mark scheme break down
- Communication skills 20%
- Knowledge 80%

Instructions for actor
You are a 40-year-old man who wears glasses. Tonight, after driving home from work in the dark, you had a sudden onset of pain in your right eye, blurring of vision, and watery eye. You have noticed it is very painful to look at the bright lights in the ED. You have not had any previous episodes. When you are examined, you cannot see normally out of the eye, even with your glasses on (reduced visual acuity), and shining light in your left eye causes pain in your right eye.

Instructions for examiner
Two minutes from the end of the station, stop the candidate and ask them 'What would your management of this patient be?'

Equipment required
Visual acquity chart
Fundoscopy
Pen torch

Curriculum mapping
Sections of the CEM (2010) curriculum relevant to this question include the following.

Common competencies
CC1 History taking
CC2 Clinical examination
CC3 Therapeutics and safe prescribing
CC4 Time management and decision-making
CC5 Decision-making and clinical reasoning
CC6 Patient as the central focus of care
CC12 Relationship with patients and communication

ACCS Acute presentations CT1&2
CAP23 Pain management
CAP29 Red eye

Mark scheme

Introduces self	1
Makes focused review of history	1
Asks about past medical history—e.g. glaucoma, cataracts, inflammatory bowel disease	2
Assesses visual acuity in both eyes (+/− use of pinhole to correct refractive errors)	2
Measures acuity from correct distance away from chart	1
Assesses visual fields	1
Assesses eye movements	1
Assesses pupil reactions—simple	1
Assesses pupil reactions—relative afferent pupil defect	1
Discusses/explains lid eversion	1
Carries out fundoscopy:	
• Correct setting up of ophthalmoscope	1
• Looks for red reflex	1
• Examines four quadrants, macula, and fovea of retina	1
• Assesses conjunctiva	1
• Assesses sclera	1
Considers and explains potential diagnosis of acute angle closure glaucoma	1
Treats with 2% pilocarpine drops, 1 drop every 15 minutes	2
Applies to **both** eyes	1
Offers analgesia	1
Organises ophthalmology review (urgent)	1
Global score from actor	5
Global score from examiner	5
Total	**33**

Question 38 Shortness of breath 2

Instructions for candidate
You are called to resus to see a 35-year-old woman who is 38 weeks pregnant and has presented in extremis with SOB. You have an experienced nurse from the ED with you. Please assess the patient and treat as necessary.

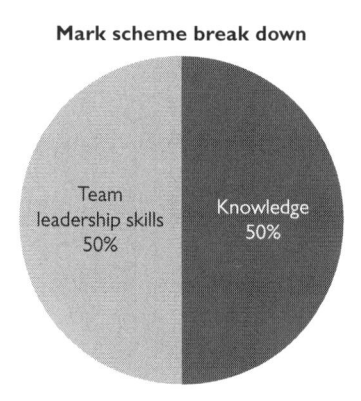

Mark scheme break down

- Team leadership skills 50%
- Knowledge 50%

Instructions for actor 1 (patient)
You are a woman who is 38 weeks pregnant. You have been well throughout the pregnancy and have no medical problems. You have become suddenly very out of breath in the last 2 hours. You are terrified that you are going to die and the baby will die too. You are very distressed.

When the candidate assesses you, you can barely speak because you are so breathless. Within a minute of starting the station, you should simulate cardiac arrest—the candidate will then use a manikin for the remainder of the station.

Instructions for actor 2 (nurse)
You are a staff nurse in the ED. You know where all the equipment is kept and can hand it to the candidate, but you don't act without being clearly instructed to do so.

Instructions for examiner
You may provide the candidate with the following information if requested:

Pulse = 160
BP = 80/40
CRT = 4 seconds
Oxygen saturations (SaO_2) = 80% on air, 93% on high-flow O_2
GCS 15
Blood glucose = 10

The patient became acutely short of breath 2 hours ago and is only able to speak in short sentences. Within a minute of the start of the station, the patient collapses into pulseless electrical activity (PEA) cardiac arrest and remains in cardiac arrest until the end of the station.

Please make sure that the candidate uses the manikin as soon as cardiac arrest is diagnosed. In the last minute of the scenario, the candidate should be advised that the obstetric consultant and ED consultant have arrived, and the candidate should give them a brief handover of the situation, indicating the need for immediate section.

Equipment required

Standard adult resuscitation equipment (see introductory section)
Delivery kit
Neonatal resuscitation kit

Curriculum mapping

Sections of the CEM (2010) curriculum relevant to this question include the following.

Common competencies

CC1 History taking
CC2 Clinical examination
CC3 Therapeutics and safe prescribing
CC4 Time management and decision-making
CC5 Decision-making and clinical reasoning
CC6 Patient as the central focus of care
CC7 Prioritization of patient safety in clinical practice
CC8 Team work and patient safety
CC12 Relationship with patients and communication
CC13 Breaking bad news
CC15 Communication with colleagues and cooperation

ACCS Major presentations CT1&2

CMP2 Cardiorespiratory arrest
CMP5 Shocked patient

ACCS Acute presentations CT1&2

CAP6 Breathlessness
CAP35 Ventilatory support

Guidelines

http://www.resus.org.uk/pages/alsalgo.pdf

http://www.rcog.org.uk/womens-health/clinical-guidance/maternal-collapse-pregnancy-and-puerperium-green-top-56

Mark scheme

Gives oxygen	1
Follows A B C D E approach	2
Asks patient to sit up or left lateral tilt	2
Calls for urgent anaesthetic and obstetric assistance	2
Measures blood glucose	1
Promptly diagnoses cardiac arrest	1
Immediately after cardiac arrest recognized, considers perimortem caesarean section within 5 minutes of starting CPR	3
Calls for urgent neonatal assistance	1

Continued

Question 38 Shortness of breath 2

Continued

Carries out early intubation	2
Provides prompt CPR	1
Gives adrenaline	1
Considers hypothermia, hypoxia, hypotension, hypo/hyperkalaemia ('4 Hs') and tamponade (cardiac), tension pneumothorax, toxins, thromboembolic ('4 Ts')	2
Maintains left lateral tilt during CPR or ensures uterine displacement to left	1
Displays team leadership skills	2
Gives brief organized handover to obstetric team (situation, background, assessment, recommendation (SBAR))	2
Global score from actor	5
Global score from examiner	5
Total	**34**

Question 39 Ophthalmoscopy

Instructions for candidate
You have a third-year medical student who has asked you how to use an ophthalmoscope in a quiet 10 minutes. You have another medical student who is happy for you to use him as a patient.

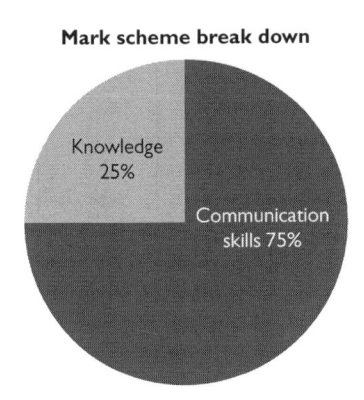

Mark scheme break down

- Knowledge 25%
- Communication skills 75%

Instructions for actor
You are a third-year medical student who is attached to the ED for the week. You have never used an ophthalmoscope before but you have seen doctors using them. You are able to follow the candidate's instructions. Do not do anything that they have not instructed you to do.

Instructions for examiner
Observation only.

Equipment required
Image of normal retina
Fundoscope
Fundoscopy model
Pen torch

Curriculum mapping
Sections of the CEM (2010) curriculum relevant to this question include the following.

Common competencies

CC2 Clinical examination
CC15 Communication with colleagues and cooperation
CC23 Teaching and training

ACCS Acute presentations CT1&2

CAP29 Red eye

Question 39 Ophthalmoscopy

Mark scheme

Explains need for fundoscopy	1
Explains what candidate should see (with aid of diagram if needed)	2
Explains some of the conditions where fundoscopy may be useful in diagnosing	1
Demonstrates the working of an ophthalmoscope including different lenses and need for different colour lenses, brightness, battery placement	2
Checks whether candidate wears glasses	1
Ensures comfort of patient (or mentions this if using model)	1
Explains technique:	
• Darkened room	1
• Explain to patient	1
• Stands to side of patient	1
• Red reflex	1
• Visualizes four quadrants	1
• Macula	1
• Fovea	1
Image of retina—correctly identifies:	
• Macula	1
• Fovea	1
• Four quadrants of retina	1
Demonstrates technique and explains what they are doing	2
Observes student performing fundoscopy and corrects technique in supportive manner	2
Encourages practice and suggests ways of gaining more skills, e.g. clinical skills lab	1
Invites questions	1
Closure—reviews learning with student	1
Global score from actor/student	5
Global score from examiner	5
Total	**39**

Question 40 Paediatric trauma

Instructions for candidate
You have a pre-alert from the ambulance service. They are on route to you from ½ a mile away with a 6-year-old boy who ran out into the street in front of a passing car. He has a reduced level of consciousness and is tachycardic. As they were so near hospital they loaded and ran. You have a paediatric nurse with you.

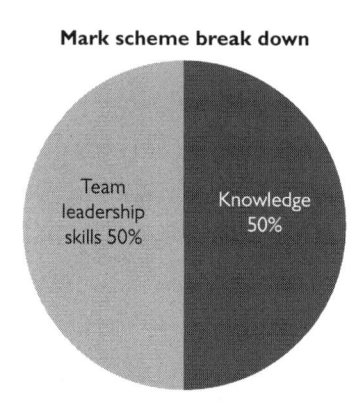

Mark scheme break down

- Team leadership skills 50%
- Knowledge 50%

Instructions for actor
You are a staff nurse who is fairly new to the ED. You know where all the equipment is kept and can hand it to the candidate, but you don't act without being clearly instructed to do so.

Instructions for examiner
When asked by the candidate, you may provide the following information:

Bruising to right side of body and leg.
A—blood and noisy gurgling respiration—will not tolerate OP airway
Collar in situ, but no blocks or tape
B—RR = 40, SaO_2 = 85% on air, 95% on O_2, reduced breath sounds to right side of chest. Flail chest on right
C—pulse = 150, CRT = 3 seconds. No IV access
D—E2, M5, V3
E—blood glucose = 6

If the candidate mentions that they are going to/would like to insert a chest drain, ask them to talk through the procedure rather than actually doing it. This will save time and reduce the need for a chest drain model.

Equipment required
Standard paediatric resuscitation equipment (see introductory section)

Curriculum mapping
Sections of the CEM (2010) curriculum relevant to this question include the following.

Question 40 Paediatric trauma

Common competencies

CC1 History taking
CC2 Clinical examination
CC4 Time management and decision-making
CC5 Decision-making and clinical reasoning
CC6 Patient as the central focus of care
CC7 Prioritization of patient safety in clinical practice
CC8 Team work and patient safety

Paediatric major presentations (PMPs)

PMP4 Major trauma in children
PMP5 Shocked child
PMP6 Unconscious child

Paediatric acute presentations (PAPs)

PAP5 Breathing difficulties—recognize the critically ill and those who will need intubation and ventilation

Guidelines available

http://www.resus.org.uk/pages/pals.pdf

Mark scheme

Calculates appropriate drug doses, weight, and tube size	3
Calls for paediatric trauma team (senior help and anaesthetist)	1
Ensures c-spine immobilization throughout	2
Administers oxygen promptly	2
Carries out suction of airway and simple airway manoeuvres	1
Recognizes need for early intubation, calls for anaesthetist if not already done so	1
Ensures intubation performed with c-spine control—directs nurse to hold neck	1
Carries out A B C D E assessment	2
Assesses breathing—RR, SaO_2, work of breathing	2
Assesses need for chest drain	1
Follows correct technique for chest drain insertion:	
• Fourth or fifth intercostal space, anterior axillary line	1
• Infiltrates with local anaesthetic	1
• Incision above rib	1
• Blunt dissection down to pleura	1
• Finger sweep inside of pleura	1
• Inserts chest tube, connects to underwater drain, secures drain in place	1
Checks bloods including blood glucose	1
Specifically requests blood products (O negative, type-specific, cross-matched blood)	1
Gives fluid bolus—10ml/kg	2
Reassesses after fluid bolus +/− 2nd 10 ml/kg	1

Continued

Continued

Assesses level of consciousness prior to anaesthesia (including pupils + GCS)	1
Summarizes findings and onward plan	1
Formulates plan including imaging—trauma series, CT scan/secondary survey	1
Shows consideration of parents	1
Displays team leadership skills	2
Global score from actor	5
Global score from examiner	5
Total	**44**

Question 41 Choking

Instructions for candidate

You are called into the resuscitation room by a nurse who is with a 2-year-old child (16 kg) who is choking on a grape. Please assess the child and manage her appropriately.

Mark scheme break down

- Team leadership skills 50%
- Knowledge 50%

Instructions for actor

You are the parent of a 2-year-old called Sarah who was eating grapes and then started coughing. You thought she was choking so you have tried slapping her on the back but you couldn't help her. So you put her in the car and came straight to hospital.

Sarah is normally fit and well, with no medical problems or allergies. You are very concerned when she suddenly becomes quiet, and want the candidate to tell you what is going on.

Instructions for examiner

Sarah is simulated by a paediatric manikin. Initially, Sarah is not coughing, but is still conscious and pink. There is no monitoring available because the child has only just arrived at hospital. The candidate should attempt to administer 5 back blows, then 5 chest thrusts.

After the candidate has done this, or after 5 minutes, you should tell the candidate 'Sarah has now gone very quiet' and when the candidate reassesses the patient, you should tell them 'She is not responding'. The candidate should then start basic life support. You may remind the candidate that the patient's weight is 16 kg. If the candidate requests monitoring of the child, this can be connected.

Observations prior to collapse:

- SaO_2 94%
- HR 130
- BP—not possible to obtain

When the child becomes unresponsive, the monitoring/defibrillator should show pulseless electrical activity. There is no response to resuscitation and no change to the clinical situation.

Equipment required

Standard paediatric resuscitation equipment (see introductory section).

Defibrillator/monitor should initially show sinus rhythm, at a rate of 130. After the patient becomes unresponsive, the rhythm changes to PEA.

Curriculum mapping

Sections of the CEM (2010) curriculum relevant to this question include the following.

Common competencies

CC1 History taking
CC2 Clinical examination
CC4 Time management and decision-making
CC12 Relationship with patients and communication
CC15 Communication with colleagues and cooperation

Paediatric major presentations (PMPs)

PMP2 Apnoea, stridor, and airway obstruction
PMP3 Cardiorespiratory arrest

Guidelines available

http://www.resus.org.uk/pages/pchkalgo.pdf

Mark scheme

Calls for ED consultant	1
Calls for paediatric and/or paediatric anaesthetist/Paediatric Intensive Care Unit (PICU)	1
Obtains a focused history:	
• Choking on grape	1
• Coughing/conscious throughout	1
Carries out assessment—does child have an effective cough?	2
Gives 5 effective back blows	2
Gives 5 effective chest thrusts	2
Reassesses	1
Recognizes and clearly states cardiac arrest	2
Puts out cardiac arrest call/paediatric resuscitation call	1
Requests resuscitation equipment including defibrillator/monitor	1
Opens airway	1
Gives 5 breaths	2
Starts CPR (score 2 for good technique)	2
Ensures monitoring connected	1
Administers adrenaline (dose 1.6 mg IV)	1
Reassesses and recognizes no response to resuscitation	1
Mentions/undertakes intubation	1
Displays team leadership skills	2
Global score from actor (parent)	5
Global score from examiner	5
Total	**36**

Question 42 Capacity

Instructions for candidate

You are looking after a 50-year-old man who presents with a massive upper gastrointestinal (GI) bleed. He his clammy, hypotensive, and tachycardic. He informs you he is a Jehovah's Witness and does not wish to have a blood transfusion. You are concerned that without blood he may die. Please discuss this with the patient.

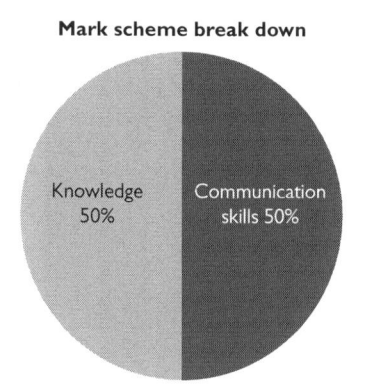

Mark scheme break down

- Knowledge 50%
- Communication skills 50%

Instructions for actor

You are a Jehovah's Witness, as are your entire family and community. No matter what the doctor says, you will not consider having blood products. You would rather die than break this rule. You understand that by refusing blood products it is possible that you will die today. You have discussed this with your wife and family previously so do not feel you need to talk to your wife about it today, but you agree to this if the doctor suggests it.

Instructions for examiner

Observation only.

Equipment required

None

Curriculum mapping

Sections of the CEM (2010) curriculum relevant to this question include the following.

Common competencies

CC1 History taking
CC3 Therapeutics and safe prescribing
CC4 Time management and decision-making
CC5 Decision-making and clinical reasoning
CC6 Patient as the central focus of care
CC7 Prioritization of patient safety in clinical practice
CC12 Relationship with patients and communication
CC13 Breaking bad news
CC15 Communication with colleagues and cooperation
CC17 Ethics and confidentiality

Self-Assessment for the MCEM Part C

CC18 Valid consent
CC19 Legal framework

ACCS Major presentations CT1&2
CMP5 Shocked patient

ACCS Acute presentations CT1&2
CAP16 Haematemesis and melaena

Mark scheme

Introduces self	1
Obtains relevant history—Jehovah's Witness	1
Explains concern about blood loss and need for blood to resuscitate	2
Explains what may happen without blood products	2
Ensures no coercion	2
Ensures patient's understanding of need for blood products	2
Allows patient opportunity to explore other options—erythropoeitin (EPO), fluids, cell saver	3
Allows patient to demonstrate that they retain the information provided—asks patient to repeat key information	1
Checks that patient believes the information provided	1
Gives patient opportunity to explain their decision—ensures patient is making an informed decision	2
Global score from examiner	5
Global score from actor	5
Total	**27**

Question 43 Limping child

Instructions for candidate
A mother has brought in her 3-year-old daughter, Laura, who has started walking with a limp over the past day. Please take a focused history and examine the child, then explain the management plan to the child's mother.

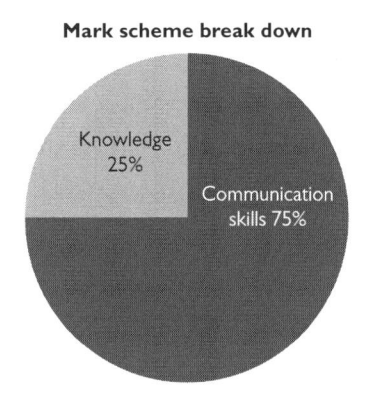

Mark scheme break down

- Knowledge 25%
- Communication skills 75%

Instructions for actor 1 (mother)
Laura has had a recent cold, which she is now recovering from. She is otherwise completely well. She has not had any recent injuries or falls and is normally well, with no medical problems, and no medications or allergies. She is immunized.

Instructions for actor 2 (child)
You have a very mild limp due to a painful right hip. You demonstrate painful rotation of the right hip, but other movements are ok.

Instructions for examiner
Observation only.

Equipment required
None.
   An adult 'actor' may be used to simulate the child if needed.

Curriculum mapping
Sections of the CEM (2010) curriculum relevant to this question include the following.

Common competencies

CC1 History taking
CC2 Clinical examination
CC4 Time management and decision-making
CC5 Decision-making and clinical reasoning
CC7 Prioritization of patient safety in clinical practice
CC12 Relationship with patients and communication

Self-Assessment for the MCEM Part C

Paediatric acute presentations (PAPs)

PAP15 Pain in children
PAP16 Painful limbs—atraumatic

Mark scheme

Introduces self	1
Obtains history of limp	1
Obtains history of fever/coryzal illness	1
Obtains history of any other joint involvement	1
Obtains history of trauma	1
Obtains history of being well/unwell	1
Asks about history around time of onset	1
Ensures child is comfortable	2
Carries out examination:	
• General inspection looking for:	3
♦ Rashes	
♦ General appearance: well/unwell	
♦ Bruises and other signs of trauma	
• Active and passive movements of both hips (flexion/extension, internal/external rotation, abduction/adduction)	2
• Tone, power, reflexes, sensation in lower limbs	2
• Observation of gait	1
Takes temperature of child	1
Recognizes that pain is localized to right hip especially on rotation of hip	2
Gives explanation of likely diagnosis—irritable hip	2
Advises no need for imaging/bloods	1
Offers treatment options—analgesia—NSAIDs, rest, gentle mobilization	2
Takes into consideration non-accidental injury (NAI)	1
Safety net—advises follow-up within 5 days, return if unwell	2
Global score from examiner	5
Global score from actor	5
Total	**38**

Question 44 Breaking bad news 3

Instructions for candidate
You are handed over a patient (a 55-year-old man) by a colleague who has gone off shift. He had arranged a CT scan of the patient's head as they had fallen over in the street, hit their head, and had a seizure. The scan showed what appears to be a large malignant-looking tumour with surrounding oedema. Please explain the scan results to the patient.

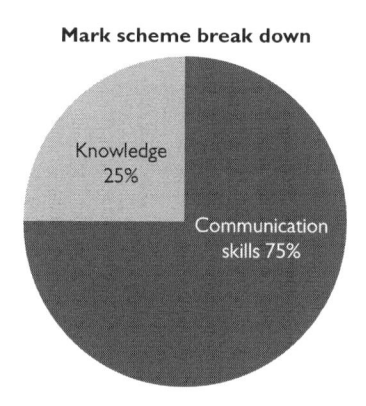

Mark scheme break down

- Knowledge 25%
- Communication skills 75%

Instructions for actor
You are a normally fit and well 55 year old, who has smoked heavily for 40 years. You have had headaches off and on over the past few weeks, but have been under stress at work. You were on your way to the bus stop after work when you collapsed to the floor and have no recollection of events until you arrived in hospital. You want to know what the scan means, what needs to be done now, and how you can be cured.

Instructions for examiner
Observation only.

Equipment required
CT scan showing a large cerebral mass, with surrounding oedema, compatible with primary brain tumour.

Curriculum mapping
Sections of the CEM (2010) curriculum relevant to this question include the following.

Common competencies

CC5 Decision-making and clinical reasoning
CC6 Patient as the central focus of care
CC12 Relationship with patients and communication
CC13 Breaking bad news

ACCS Major presentations CT1&2

CAP5 Blackout/collapse
CAP15 Fits/seizure

Self-Assessment for the MCEM Part C

Mark scheme

Introduces self to patient and explains role	2
Asks if can have nurse present, no pager/disturbances, etc.	1
Checks what has happened and what patient knows so far	2
Explains what CT scan shows	3
Explains need for further investigation to establish if appearances are due to benign or malignant, and primary or metastatic process	2
Gives patient opportunity to ask questions and answers appropriately	2
Broadly covers treatment options—for primary tumour and cerebral mets (dexamethasone, chemotherapy, radiotherapy, neurosurgical intervention)	2
Offers to call relatives/friends	1
Patient had a seizure so needs to discuss driving restrictions—if required	2
Global score from examiner	5
Global score from actor	5
Total	**27**

Question 45 Dysuria

Instructions for candidate
You are asked to see a 28-year-old man who has attended the ED complaining of dysuria for 2 days. Please take a history and explain your management plan to the patient.

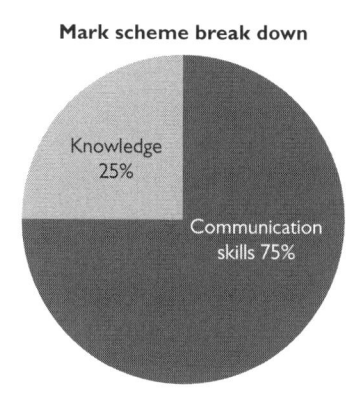

Mark scheme break down

- Knowledge 25%
- Communication skills 75%

Instructions for actor
You have been having pain on passing urine, urinary frequency, and a penile discharge for the past 2 days. On direct questioning, you have recently returned from a business trip to Thailand where you had sexual intercourse with a prostitute without using barrier protection. You have also developed bilateral knee and ankle pain.

You are not married, but have been in a relationship with a girl for the past 2 years. You don't want her to know about this 'indiscretion'. You have no medical problems, take no medication, and have no allergies. You smoke 10 cigarettes a day, occasionally smoke cannabis, but take no other drugs. You work in Information Technology for a large company.

Instructions for examiner
Observation only.

Equipment required
None

Curriculum mapping
Sections of the CEM (2010) curriculum relevant to this question include the following.

Common competencies

CC1 History taking
CC3 Therapeutics and safe prescribing
CC4 Time management and decision-making
CC5 Decision-making and clinical reasoning
CC6 Patient as the central focus of care
CC10 Infection control
CC12 Relationship with patients and communication

Mark scheme

Introduces self	1
Establishes history of dysuria	1
Establishes history of foreign travel	1
Establishes history of sexual intercourse with prostitute	2
Establishes history of not using barrier protection	1
Obtains history for joint aches	1
Asks about recent sexual history	2
Obtains past medical history (specifically):	
• Drug history	1
• Allergies	1
• Immunization history	1
Explains possibility of STI and need for self and partner testing	2
Explains probable diagnosis of Reiters disease secondary to non-gonoccocal urethritis	2
Discusses Hep B, Hep C, + HIV	2
Offers treatment options for non-specific urethritis, post-exposure prophylaxis, + Hep B vac	2
Offers generic advice:	
• Advises to complete course of antibiotics	1
• Discusses side-effects of medication	1
• Advises abstinence from sex	1
• Advises follow-up in GUM clinic	1
Global score from examiner	5
Global score from actor	5
Total	**34**

Question 46 Cranial nerve examination

Instructions for candidate
Please perform an examination of this patient's cranial nerves, naming each as you examine them.

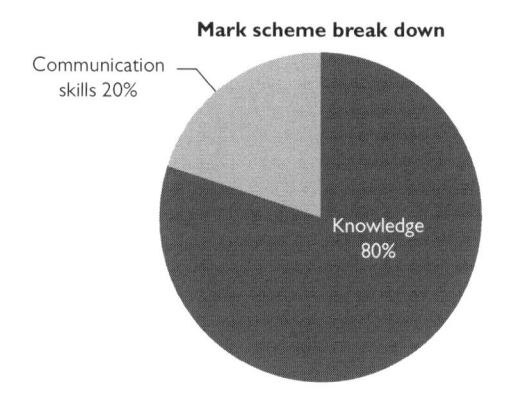

Mark scheme break down
- Communication skills 20%
- Knowledge 80%

Instructions for actor
You have a normal neurological examination.

Instructions for examiner
Observation only.

Equipment required
Cotton wool
Tendon hammer
Pins (for pinprick sensation)
Tuning fork
Tongue depressor

Curriculum mapping
Sections of the CEM (2010) curriculum relevant to this question include the following.

Common competencies
CC2 Clinical examination
CC12 Relationship with patients and communication

ACCS Major presentations CT1&2
CAP37 Weakness and paralysis

Self-Assessment for the MCEM Part C

Mark scheme

Introduces self	1
Explains examination and gains consent (verbal)	1
Assesses:	
• Olfactory (cranial nerve I)—sense of smell	1
• Eye movements—occulomotor CN III, trochlear CN IV-superior oblique (down and out), abducens CN VI-lateral rectus	2
• Visual fields—optic CN II	2
• Visual acuity—optic CN II	1
• Pupil reactions—simple, consensual, relative afferent papillary defect—optic CN II	2
• Facial sensation—trigeminal (CN V)	1
• Corneal reflex—trigeminal (CN V)	1
• Muscles of facial expression/function—facial (CN VII)	1
• Sensation to anterior two-thirds of tongue—facial (CN VII)	1
• Hearing—Webers and Rhinnes—vestibulocochlear (CN VIII)	2
Inspects uvula, sensation to posterior third of tongue, lifts uvular + checks gag reflex—glossopharyngeal (CN IX) and vagus (CN X)	2
Assesses shoulder shrug, sternocleidomastoid—accessory nerve (CN XI)	1
Assesses tongue movement—hypoglossal (CN XII)	1
Carries out examination in a systematic, organized way	2
Global score from examiner	5
Global score from actor	5
Total	**32**

Question 47 Peripheral nervous system

Instructions for candidate
This 70-year-old male patient has had a sudden onset of a left-sided weakness and left facial droop 45 minutes ago. The patient has a history of atrial fibrillation, hypertension, and high cholesterol. Please examine his peripheral neurological system.

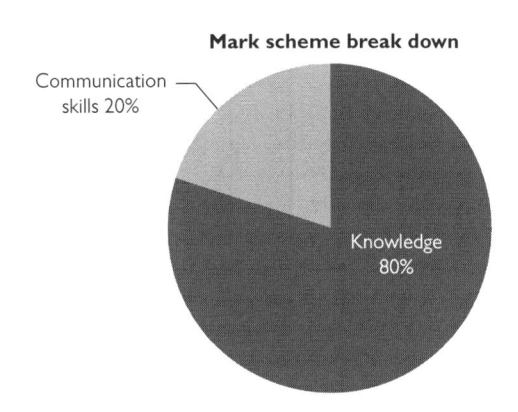

Mark scheme break down

- Communication skills 20%
- Knowledge 80%

Instructions for actor
You noticed the weakness about 45 minutes ago when you were trying to make a cup of tea in the kitchen at home. You have not had a headache and you have never had this happen before.

Your past medical history includes high cholesterol and high BP. You are on a cholesterol tablet at night, and two BP tablets and aspirin. You are not on warfarin.

You are weak down your left side, with inability to move your left arm. You can lift your left leg with difficulty and cannot keep it raised off the bed for 5 seconds. If you try to blow out your cheeks, air leaks from the left side of your mouth, and you have been dribbling from the left side of your mouth.

Instructions for examiner
Observation only.

Equipment required
Tendon hammer
Cotton wool
Tuning fork

Curriculum mapping
Sections of the CEM (2010) curriculum relevant to this question include the following.

Common competencies
CC2 Clinical examination
CC12 Relationship with patients and communication

ACCS Major presentations CT1&2
CAP37 Weakness and paralysis

Self-Assessment for the MCEM Part C

Mark scheme

Introduces self	1
Explains examination and gains consent (verbal)	1
Examines upper limb:	
• Appearance	1
• Tone	1
• Power	1
• Reflex	1
• Sensation	1
• Coordination	1
Examines lower limb:	
• Appearance	1
• Tone	1
• Power	1
• Reflex	1
• Sensation	1
• Coordination	1
Assesses gait	1
Carries out examination in a systematic, organized way	2
Summarizes findings	2
Makes diagnosis	1
Suggests management plan	1
Global score from examiner	5
Global score from actor	5
Total	**31**

Question 48 Ankle plaster

Instructions for candidate
This 35-year-old woman has fallen down some steps in a nightclub. She has a comminuted fracture of her distal tibia and distal fibula. She is going to have an operation on it in the next 24 hours. Please apply an appropriate plaster for this injury. You have one untrained assistant.

Mark scheme break down

- Communication skills 20%
- Knowledge 30%
- Practical skills 50%

Instructions for actor 1 (patient)
You have fallen down a couple of steps when leaving a nightclub. You landed badly on your left ankle and have got severe pain in the outside of the ankle. You have already been told it is broken and that you need an operation.

Allow the candidate to put a plaster on. Any movement or touching of the ankle causes you severe pain.

Instructions for actor 2 (assistant)
You have not done this task before. You are able to follow instructions when given.

Instructions for examiner
Observation only.

Equipment required
Plaster kit
Appropriate X-ray

Curriculum mapping
Sections of the CEM (2010) curriculum relevant to this question include the following.

Common competencies

CC2 Clinical examination
CC3 Therapeutics and safe prescribing
CC4 Time management and decision-making
CC5 Decision-making and clinical reasoning
CC6 Patient as the central focus of care
CC7 Prioritization of patient safety in clinical practice

CC8 Team work and patient safety
CC9 Principles of safety and quality improvement
CC10 Infection control
CC12 Relationship with patients and communication
CC18 Valid consent

ACCS Acute presentations CT1&2

CAP23 Pain management
CAP33 Traumatic limb and joint injuries

Mark scheme

Introduces self/confirms identity of patient	1
Asks about analgesia/offers analgesia—considers entonox	1
Explains need for plaster + reviews X-rays with patient	1
Ensures correct position of patient	2
Measures plaster	1
Applies correct thickness of plaster	1
Applies Tubinette™/gauze layers	1
Demonstrates correct placement of backslab	2
Secures with bandage	1
Ensures no rough edges	1
Plaster covers from back of knee to metatarsal-phalangeal joints (MTPJs)	2
Applies plaster stirrup	1
Moulds plaster with ankle in dorsiflexion	1
Checks distal neurovascular supply	1
Obtains check X-ray	1
Considers extending plaster above knee	1
Mentions/applies elevation	1
Advises about plaster—getting wet, risk of soft tissue swelling, etc.	2
Invites questions	1
Global score from examiner	5
Global score from actor	5
Total	**33**

Question 49 Wrist examination

Instructions for candidate
This 65-year-old woman tripped over on the way back home from the shops and injured her right wrist. She was sent to X-ray from triage. Please assess the patient with her X-ray and explain the management required.

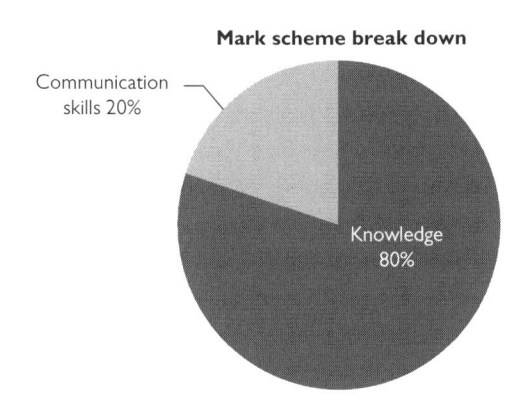

Mark scheme break down
- Communication skills 20%
- Knowledge 80%

Instructions for actor
You are a 65-year-old woman who tripped over on uneven pavement this morning while shopping. You have no medical problems and are right handed. When the candidate examines you, your right wrist is extremely painful. You think your wrist looks bent out of shape.

You have no previous medical illnesses. On examination you have a severely deformed wrist, with reduced sensation in medial nerve distribution. The candidate should explain to you that the wrist is badly broken, and that one of the nerves that supplies the hand has been injured. They should explain that the wrist needs to be manipulated and put in plaster.

Instructions for examiner
Observation only.

Equipment required
X-ray image of displaced distal radius fracture

Curriculum mapping
Sections of the CEM (2010) curriculum relevant to this question include the following.

Common competencies

CC2 Clinical examination
CC4 Time management and decision-making
CC5 Decision-making and clinical reasoning
CC6 Patient as the central focus of care
CC7 Prioritization of patient safety in clinical practice
CC12 Relationship with patients and communication
CC18 Valid consent

ACCS Acute presentations CT1&2
CAP23 Pain management
CAP33 Traumatic limb and joint injuries

Mark scheme

Introduces self	1
Offers analgesia	1
Asks about mechanism of injury	1
Asks about history of falls	1
Examines upper limb from clavicle to wrist	2
Examines median, ulnar, and radial nerve distribution + digital nerves	2
Checks vascular supply	1
Reviews X-ray and explains fracture to patient	2
Explains need for manipulation as neurological compromise (median nerve)	2
Explains need for written consent	1
Explains procedure and appropriate sedation or regional anaesthesia	2
Ensures no contraindications to chosen procedure	2
Global score from examiner	5
Global score from actor	5
Total	**27**

Question 50 Handover

Instructions for candidate

You have come in for the late shift in your ED. All your major end bays are full, but you have three empty beds on the observation unit. You need to do a 'board round' of the patients in Majors and decide on provisional allocation of these patients with the nurse in charge. The information about each patient is provided in Table 2.1.

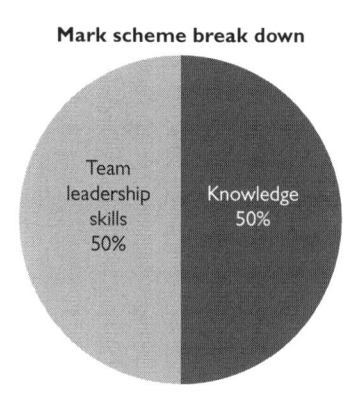

Mark scheme break down

- Team leadership skills 50%
- Knowledge 50%

Instructions for actor

You are the nurse in charge of a busy shift in the ED. Your registrar wants to go through the patients to improve patient flow. Please allow the candidate to go through the white board, without making any suggestions, but agree to their plan.

Table 2.1 Information on each patient

Bay	Patient	Working diagnosis	Plan
1	68-year-old male	Renal colic	Obs ward for CTKUB in morning
2	35-year-old female	Musculoskeletal lower back pain and urine retention	Analgesia, mobilize, home
3	82-year-old male	Collapse in nursing home? #NOF	Ortho bed requested. In X-ray
4	19-year-old female	RIF pain	? Appendicitis, Obs ward awaiting surgical bed
5	48-year-old male	#Tib and fib	
6	80-year-old male	Fall down stairs, ongoing neck pain. Normal plain X-rays	Analgesia, mobilize
7	60-year-old female	# Left wrist for manipulation under Bier's block	Awaiting manipulation
8	40-year-old male	Panic attack—2/52 post removal of plaster for # tibia	Home
9	55-year-old male	Alcoholic. Vomiting f or 3 days. Tachypnoea. ?Alcohol withdrawal	Home
10	28-year-old female	OD of dothiepin—sleepy	Obs for psych review in morning

Abbreviations: # fracture; CTKUB computerized topography scan of kidney, ureters, and bladder; NOF neck of femur; Obs ward Observation ward; OD overdose; ortho orthopaedic; psych psychiatry; RIF right iliac fossa.

Self-Assessment for the MCEM Part C

If asked for more details about each patient, you can say that you have just arrived on shift and haven't had a handover yet, as your colleague has been called away to help in resus for 5 minutes (see Table 2.1).

Instructions for examiner
Observation only.

The candidate should be allowed to see Table 2.1 during the 1-minute preparation for the station, and throughout the station.

Equipment required
Copy of ward sheet per candidate

Curriculum mapping
Sections of the CEM (2010) curriculum relevant to this question include the following.

Common competencies

CC1 History taking
CC4 Time management and decision-making
CC5 Decision-making and clinical reasoning
CC6 Patient as the central focus of care
CC7 Prioritization of patient safety in clinical practice
CC8 Team work and patient safety
CC9 Principles of safety and quality improvement
CC10 Infection control
CC15 Communication with colleagues and cooperation
CC23 Teaching and training

Mark scheme

Bay 1—need to consider abdominal aortic aneurysm (AAA). Either focused assessment with sonography for trauma (FAST) scan/CT aorta or admit under surgeons	2
Bay 2—cauda equina—required emergency MRI spine	2
Bay 3—need to consider cause of collapse and dependence of patient for observation unit	2
Bay 4—has a pregnancy test been done? Not to observation unit before negative beta human chorionic gonadotrophin (BHCG)	2
Bay 5—await orthopaedic bed—could go to observation unit to await bed if needed as long as neurovascularly intact + plaster applied	2
Bay 6—unable to clinically clear cervical spine if ongoing pain. Needs to remain immobilized until CT of c-spine can be undertaken	2
Bay 7—could wait on observation unit for manipulation if neurovascularly intact + plaster applied + mechanical fall only	2
Bay 8—? pulmonary embolism (PE). Has appropriate investigation been undertaken before labelling as panic attack?	2
Bay 9—needs venous blood gas (VBG) in case of alcoholic ketoacidosis	2
Bay 10—tricyclic overdose. If still drowsy needs cardiac monitoring. ? if appropriate for observation unit	2
Demonstrates systematic, organized approach	2
Global score from examiner	5
Global score from actor	5
Total	**32**

Question 51 Elbow injury

Instructions for candidate
Please apply a plaster of Paris to this patient with a left-sided undisplaced olecranon fracture.

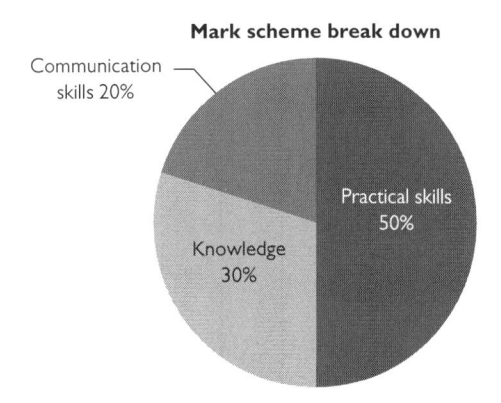

Mark scheme break down
- Communication skills 20%
- Practical skills 50%
- Knowledge 30%

Instructions for actor
Your elbow is extremely painful. You can bend it slowly to get into the position the candidate shows you. Follow the instructions from the candidate.

Instructions for examiner
Observation only.

Equipment required
Plaster kit
X-ray

Curriculum mapping
Sections of the CEM (2010) curriculum relevant to this question include the following.

Common competencies

CC2 Clinical examination
CC7 Prioritization of patient safety in clinical practice
CC12 Relationship with patients and communication

ACCS Acute presentations CT1&2

CAP23 Pain management
CAP33 Traumatic limb and joint injuries

Self-Assessment for the MCEM Part C

Mark scheme

Introduces self	1
Considers patient's pain throughout procedure	1
Explains procedure and obtains verbal consent	2
Checks X-ray	1
Checks neurovascular status	1
Applies Velband® to skin	2
Cuts plaster length from wrist to just distal to deltoid	2
Ensures appropriate water temperature	1
Cuts plaster to shape	2
Applies plaster to radial border of forearm and lateral border of upper arm	2
Bandages in place	2
Provides sling	1
Gives appropriate advice post plaster of Paris + symptoms that would be of concern	2
Arranges and explains follow-up	1
Global score from examiner	5
Global score from actor	5
Total	**31**

Question 52 Airway management

Instructions for candidate

You have had a pre-alert from the ambulance service. They are bringing you a 40-year-old man who collapsed at home after complaining about a thunderclap headache. He was initially combative, but has progressively become less responsive. Please assess him and manage as appropriate. You have an ED nurse to help you.

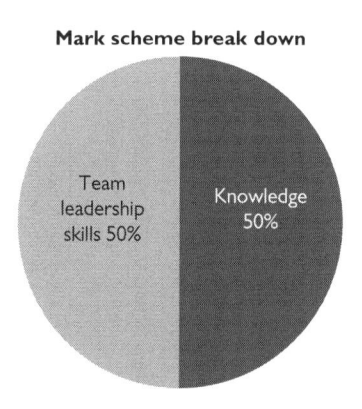

Mark scheme break down

- Team leadership skills 50%
- Knowledge 50%

Instructions for actor

You are a very new ED nurse. Only act on instruction from the candidate. You do not have any advanced airway skills.

Instructions for examiner

The ITU anaesthetist is busy on unit. When asked by the candidate, you may provide the following information:

A—partially obstructive, gurgling ventilation—needs OP/NP airways
B—RR = 18, SaO_2 = 95% on air, will tolerate airway adjuncts
C—pulse = 45, BP = 200/105
D—E2, V2, M4, pupils left = 3 mm, right = 6 mm
E—blood glucose = 6
Estimated weight = 70 kg

The patient requires rapid sequence induction of anaesthesia (RSI) using appropriate drugs and appropriate monitoring. No marks are added or deducted for use of appropriate opiate (fentanyl or alfentanil).

Equipment required

Standard adult resuscitation equipment (see introductory section)
Intubating manikin

Curriculum mapping

Sections of the CEM (2010) curriculum relevant to this question include the following.

Self-Assessment for the MCEM Part C

Common competencies

CC1 History taking
CC2 Clinical examination
CC3 Therapeutics and safe prescribing
CC4 Time management and decision-making
CC5 Decision-making and clinical reasoning
CC6 Patient as the central focus of care
CC7 Prioritization of patient safety in clinical practice
CC8 Team work and patient safety
CC15 Communication with colleagues and cooperation

ACCS Major presentations CT1&2

CMP6 Unconscious patient

ACCS Acute presentations CT1&2

CAP5 Blackout/collapse
CAP17 Headache

Mark scheme

Calls for anaesthetic help	1
Gives oxygen by facemask	1
Follows simple airway opening manoeuvres	1
Uses airway adjuncts—OP/NP airways	
• Correctly sized	1
Suctions oropharynx	1
Assesses breathing and circulation and blood glucose before anaesthesia	2
Selects appropriate induction agent—propofol or thiopentone and appropriate dose (100–200 mg propofol, 300–400 mg thiopentone)	1
Gives appropriate dose of suxamethonium (70–150 mg)	1
Vasopressor drawn up pre-RSI—metoraminol or ephedrine	1
Pre-oxygenates for 3 minutes—using BVM	2
Appropriately monitors non-invasive blood pressure (NIBP), SaO_2, ECG, $ETCO_2$ (1/2 mark for each)	2
Uses appropriate equipment—size 3 or 4 Mackintosh blade, size 8 or 9 oral endotracheal tube (OETT), tape	1
Rescues airway—using LMA	1
Demonstrates appropriate RSI technique	2
Confirms OETT position using $ETCO_2$ and stethoscope	1
Considers mannitol or hypertonic saline	1
Appropriately images CXR (tube position) and CT head	2
Demonstrates team leadership skills	2
Global score from examiner	5
Global score from actor	5
Total	**35**

Question 53 Sedation

Instructions for candidate
You have been asked to speak to the mother of Joseph, a 3-year-old boy, who has fallen and cut his top lip. The wound needs suturing, and your consultant has suggested ketamine sedation to facilitate this. He has asked you to explain the process to Joseph's mother, check Joseph is a suitable candidate for sedation, and get her to sign a consent form.

Mark scheme break down

- Knowledge 25%
- Communication skills 75%

Instructions for actor
You are the single mother of 3-year-old Joseph. He has fallen on the trampoline in your back garden and banged his lip on the frame of the trampoline. He has a small cut to the centre of his upper lip, which looks awful. You called an ambulance immediately. You saw it happen and were in the garden with him at the time.

Jo has not eaten since breakfast 4 hours ago. He has no medical problems, takes no medications, and his immunizations are up to date. He has been to hospital once before, when he was 18 months old and fell over in the kitchen. He cut his left eyebrow, which was sorted out with skin glue. The staff in the ED wrapped him up in a blanket to stop him struggling, in order to put the glue on. You are not very keen to agree to ketamine sedation because you have heard all about ketamine being used as a street drug. You have read a newspaper article about long-term bladder problems with ketamine. The candidate should ask you why you are reluctant, and explore your concerns.

Initially, you request that the procedure is done by wrapping Jo up in a blanket. If you are offered reassurance, and a clear explanation, you agree to sign the consent form for ketamine sedation.

Instructions for examiner
Observation only.

Equipment required
None

Curriculum mapping
Sections of the CEM (2010) curriculum relevant to this question include the following.

Common competencies

CC1 History taking
CC3 Therapeutics and safe prescribing
CC6 Patient as the central focus of care

CC7 Prioritization of patient safety in clinical practice
CC8 Team work and patient safety
CC12 Relationship with patients and communication
CC18 Valid consent

Paediatric acute presentations (PAPs)

PAP15 Pain in children
PAP17 Painful limbs—traumatic

Guidelines available

http://www.collemergencymed.ac.uk/shop-floor/Clinical%20Guidelines/College%20Guidelines/, then follow **Safe Sedation in the Emergency Department**

Mark scheme

Introduces self, checks mother's identity	1
Uses open question to start	1
Asks what mother understands so far/recaps situation	1
Adequately explains procedure:	
• Sedation to allow adequate suturing	1
• Suturing recommended for this type/site of injury (involving vermillion border)	1
• Need for IV access	1
• What to expect during sedation, e.g. emergency phenomena, movements	1
Consideration of alternatives:	
• Wrap—poor cosmetic result as likely to move	1
• Entonox—no access to mouth	1
• Formal general anaesthesia (GA)—night in hospital	1
Checks contra-indications to sedation:	
• Previous problems with GA	1
• Full stomach	1
• Recent illnesses	1
• Allergies	1
Explains plan for recovery from sedation	1
Gives advice about discharge from hospital	1
Invites questions	1
Addresses concerns/answers questions	1
Explains need for consent form	1
Includes the following when gaining informed consent:	1
• Wound problems, e.g. infection	1
• Sedation problems, e.g. emergency phenomena, vomiting	1
Global score from examiner	5
Global score from actor	5
Total	**32**

Question 54 Neck injury 2

Instructions for candidate
This patient was the front-seat passenger in a rear-end shunt. The patient has been 'collared and boarded' by the ambulance crew. Please assess the patient, remove them safely from the spinal board, and explain your ongoing management.

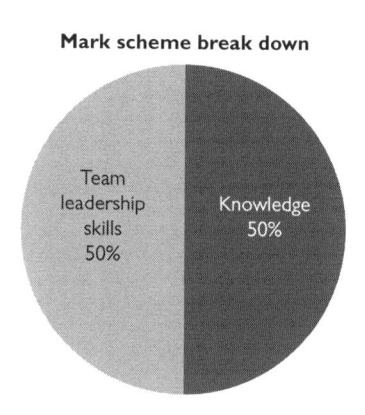

Mark scheme break down

- Team leadership skills 50%
- Knowledge 50%

Instructions for actor
You have been involved in a car accident earlier today. You were in the passenger seat of your friend's car, waiting at traffic lights, when another car, at low speed, shunted the back of your car.

You and the driver were wearing your seatbelts and were not injured significantly. You got out of the car to see if there was any damage to the car, and someone else called an ambulance. When the ambulance arrived, the paramedics made you lie down by the side of the road, and they put a collar on your neck and laid you on a hard board. You have been lying on the board for an hour now, and your neck and back are starting to get a bit stiff all over. You still have no pain anywhere. You have no weakness or abnormal sensation.

You were on your way to work in a shop when the car crashed into you. You have not had any drugs or alcohol today, and you are not confused. You have no medical problems and take no medication. You are cooperative when the candidate asks you questions and examines you.

Instructions for examiner
Observation only.
Four other helpers will be required to take part in the log roll.

Equipment required
Cervical collar
'Sand bags'
Tape
Tendon hammer
Pen torch

Curriculum mapping
Sections of the CEM (2010) curriculum relevant to this question include the following.

Common competencies

CC1 History taking
CC2 Clinical examination
CC5 Decision-making and clinical reasoning
CC6 Patient as the central focus of care
CC7 Prioritization of patient safety in clinical practice
CC8 Team work and patient safety
CC12 Relationship with patients and communication
CC15 Communication with colleagues and cooperation

ACCS Acute presentations CT1&2

CAP21 Neck pain
CAP23 Pain management

Guidelines available

http://www.collemergencymed.ac.uk/shop-floor/Clinical%20Guidelines/College%20Guidelines/, then follow **Cervical Spine: Management of Alert, Adult Patients with Potential Cervical Spine Injury in the Emergency Department**

Mark scheme

Introduces self	1
Uses open question to start, e.g. 'Tell me what happened'	1
Explains reason for lying on hard board with collar on—need to assess injuries	1
Checks details of mechanism of injury:	
• Low speed	1
• Rear shunt	1
Checks injuries sustained	1
Asks about neck pain and back pain	1
Asks about neurological symptoms	1
Asks about alcohol or drugs	1
Checks orientation	1
Asks about driver of car	1
Carries out brief neurological assessment of upper and lower limbs	1
Undertakes log roll:	
• Explains log roll adequately to patient	1
• Gathers team for log roll—uses four people	1
• Checks team know technique of log roll	1
• Instructs team	1
• Examines all areas of spine	1
• Examines back of head	1
• Removes spinal board safely	1
Removes cervical spine collar:	
• Explains adequately to patient, e.g. keep head still	1

Continued

Question 54 Neck injury 2

Continued

• Ensures collar undone with manual inline stabilization	1
• Palpates cervical spine	1
• Assesses rotation	1
Decides to remove collar	2
Does not request imaging	1
Explains to patient:	
• No evidence of significant injury	1
• Analgesia advice	1
• Mobilization advice	1
• Natural history of soft tissue neck injury (whiplash)	1
Demonstrates team leadership skills	2
Global score from examiner	5
Global score from actor	5
Total	**42**

Question 55 Seizure 1

Instructions for candidate

This patient has been brought to the ED after collapsing at work. His colleagues have described to the ambulance crew that he was sitting at his desk when he suddenly slumped in his chair and began jerking his arms and legs, so they phoned 999.

This has never happened before. Please take a history and explain to the patient what will happen next.

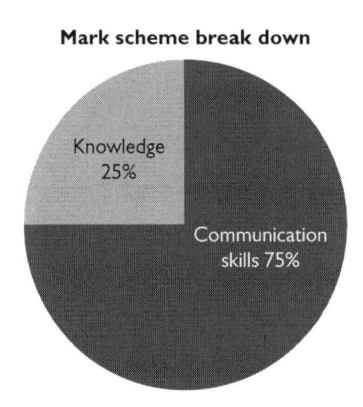

Mark scheme break down

- Knowledge 25%
- Communication skills 75%

Instructions for actor

You have had your first epileptic seizure today at work. You can't remember much about it. You remember sitting at your desk, feeling absolutely fine, and making a few phone calls, before it happened. When you 'came round' you were lying on the floor at work, with lots of people looking at you, and the paramedics arrived shortly afterwards and brought you to hospital. You had been incontinent. You can't remember what happened during your seizure but the paramedics have told you it looked like an epileptic seizure.

You were completely well until this happened. You have no medical problems, take no medication, and have not been ill recently. You have not had any recent head injuries. You drink alcohol moderately— 'a few beers, or glasses of wine, twice a week'—you have never been a heavy drinker, and never use drugs. You are active and regularly go to the gym and play 5-aside football with friends. Your older brother has epilepsy and has been on medication for years. Your work is office based and involves administration for a large company. You have a driving licence but you don't own a car and you walk to work.

You are happy to go along with anything the candidate recommends, in terms of investigations and recommendations about staying in hospital, or going home. You have a good GP who you would be happy to go and see about this.

Instructions for examiner

Observation only.

Equipment required

None

Curriculum mapping

Sections of the CEM (2010) curriculum relevant to this question include the following.

Question 55 Seizure 1

Common competencies

CC1 History taking
CC5 Decision-making and clinical reasoning
CC6 Patient as the central focus of care
CC7 Prioritization of patient safety in clinical practice
CC12 Relationship with patients and communication

ACCS Acute presentations CT1&2

CAP5 Blackout/collapse
CAP15 Fits/seizure

Guidelines available

http://www.collemergencymed.ac.uk/shop-floor/Clinical%20Guidelines/College%20Guidelines/, then follow **First Seizure in the ED**

Mark scheme

Introduces self	1
Uses open question to start, e.g. 'Tell me what happened'	1
Asks about past history of seizures	1
Prior to the seizure asks about:	
• Warning signs (prodromal symptoms)	1
• What exactly was patient doing prior to fit	1
• Recent illness/new symptoms	1
• Head injury	1
• Alcohol or drug use	1
During the seizure asks about:	
• Memory of events	1
• Length of seizure	1
• Description from colleagues—type of movements	1
• Incontinence or tongue biting	1
After the seizure asks about:	
• How long to return to normal	1
• Tired/drowsy/post-ictal	1
• Injuries sustained	1
Obtains past medical history:	
• Alcohol intake	1
• Drug intake	1
• Medical problems	1
Obtains family history	1
Obtains social history, e.g. job	1
Explains to patient:	
• Need for examination	1

Continued

Self-Assessment for the MCEM Part C

Continued

• Basic investigations, e.g. ECG, blood glucose	1
• If examination and investigations normal—first fit clinic	2
• If abnormalities found in examination or investigations, may need additional tests and/or to stay in hospital	2
• No driving + inform Driver and Vehicle Licensing Agency (DVLA)	1
Invites questions	1
Global score from examiner	5
Global score from actor	5
Total	**40**

Question 56 Regional anaesthesia 1

Instructions for candidate
This woman has tripped over the pavement and sustained a displaced Colles fracture, which needs to be manipulated and immobilized. You have decided to use regional IV anaesthesia (Bier's block) to facilitate this, which is standard practice in your ED. Please explain the procedure to the patient and gain her consent. You are not expected to perform the procedure.

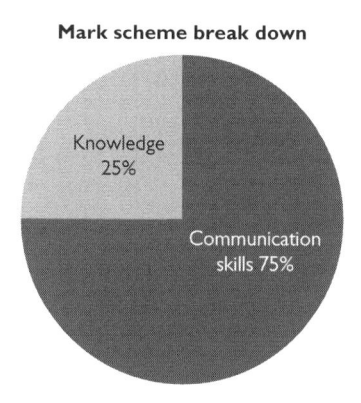

Mark scheme break down

- Knowledge 25%
- Communication skills 75%

Instructions for actor
You are a 78-year-old woman who has tripped over in town while you were doing your shopping. You have broken your right wrist. You have no other injuries. You were brought to hospital by ambulance after someone in the street phoned 999. You have been seen by a triage nurse, who told you that your wrist is probably broken. You were given some paracetamol tablets and sent for an X-ray. The person who took your X-ray says your wrist is broken and it's quite a bad break.

You live with your husband and, usually, you're quite independent—you don't have any home help and you both drive the car. You're right handed. You have high BP and a history of bowel cancer several years ago, but you have had an operation and been given the all clear.

Instructions for examiner
Observation only.

Equipment required
None

Curriculum mapping
Sections of the CEM (2010) curriculum relevant to this question include the following.

Common competencies
CC1 History taking
CC6 Patient as the central focus of care
CC7 Prioritization of patient safety in clinical practice
CC12 Relationship with patients and communication
CC18 Valid consent

ACCS Acute presentations CT1&2
CAP23 Pain management
CAP33 Traumatic limb and joint injuries

Guidelines available

http://www.collemergencymed.ac.uk/shop-floor/clinicalguidelines/, then follow **Intravenous Regional Anaesthesia for Distal Forearm Fractures (Bier's Block)**

Mark scheme

Introduces self	1
Explains diagnosis—displaced wrist fracture	1
Explains need to be manipulated to allow healing	2
Checks circumstances of fall:	
• Establishes mechanical fall	1
• No preceding symptoms	1
• Checks no other injuries	1
Explains plan for procedure under regional anaesthesia	1
Explains procedure:	
• Move to a monitored bed/resus bed	1
• ECG	1
• Cannula in both hands	1
• Double inflatable tight cuff around upper arm	1
• Inject local anaesthetic	1
• Allow to work	1
• Manipulate fracture	1
• Apply plaster	1
• Repeat X-ray	1
• If position of fracture adequate, remove cuff after 20 minutes	1
Checks contra-indications:	
• Severe hypertension	1
• Allergy to local anaesthetic	1
• Majority of: other injuries to same arm, methaemoglobinaemia, sickle cell disease, infected limb, epilepsy, Raynaud's phenomenom	1
Explains risks:	
• Failure to achieve adequate position—may require surgery	1
• Failure of technique to provide adequate analgesia	1
• Allergic reaction	1
Explains other options, e.g. plaster without manipulation, or straight to surgery	1
Checks patient will cope at home after the procedure with arm in plaster	1
Explains post-procedure management:	
• Home	1

Continued

Continued

• Analgesia	1
• Fracture clinic	1
Invites questions	1
Global score from examiner	5
Global score from actor	5
Total	**40**

Question 57 Ankle injury

Instructions for candidate
This patient has ankle pain after sustaining an inversion injury. She has had some paracetamol and come into the 'Minor injuries' part of the ED to be seen.

Please take a focused history, examine the patient's ankle, and advise them about management.

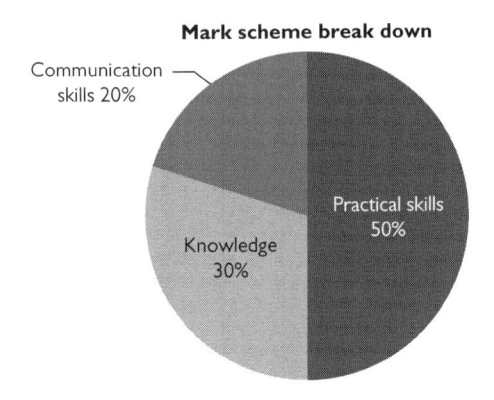

Mark scheme break down
- Communication skills 20%
- Knowledge 30%
- Practical skills 50%

Instructions for actor
You are a 19-year-old woman who has a painful ankle after twisting it last night. You were out with some friends, having a few drinks in the local pub, and when you came to go home you jumped down the pub steps. You landed awkwardly on your right ankle but were able to walk the rest of the way home. This morning it was still sore so you have come to the ED to get an X-ray.

You have mild asthma and you are just on salbutamol inhalers, and no other medication. You have taken ibuprofenbefore and it doesn't make you wheezy.

You are a student, currently living at home with your parents. You play netball for your college and have a match next week. You don't usually drink very much alcohol. Last night was your best friend's birthday and you had too much to drink. Normally, you only have 2–3 drinks on a night out.

When the candidate examines you, you are tender 'all over' but nowhere specifically hurts more than any other place. You are able to walk, but it feels painful when you put weight through your ankle or move it. You are keen to have an X-ray and keep asking for one, even if the candidate tells you it's not necessary. If the candidate doesn't advise you about return to sport, you should ask when you can play netball again.

Instructions for examiner
Observation only.

Equipment required
None

Curriculum mapping
Sections of the CEM (2010) curriculum relevant to this question include the following.

Common competencies

CC1 History taking
CC2 Clinical examination

Question 57 Ankle injury

CC3 Therapeutics and safe prescribing
CC4 Time management and decision-making
CC5 Decision-making and clinical reasoning
CC6 Patient as the central focus of care
CC11 Management of long-term conditions and promoting patient self-care

ACCS Acute presentations CT1&2

CAP23 Pain management
CAP33 Traumatic limb and joint injuries

Mark scheme

Introduces self	1
Takes history:	
• Exact mechanism of injury, e.g. inversion or eversion	1
• Weight bearing	1
• Other injuries	1
Takes past medical history, medications	1
Carries out examination:	
• Offers analgesia	1
• Gait	1
• Inspection of both ankles	1
• Thorough palpation of ankle joint, including proximal fibula	2
• Movements—dorsi/plantar flexion, eversion, inversion	2
• Neurovascular assessment	1
Explains:	
• Likely to be a soft tissue injury	1
• No X-ray required	1
When challenged states no imaging required and why. Discusses Ottawa ankle rules including:	
• If no tenderness at distal 6 cm of posterior medial malleolus and lateral malleolus	1
• Weight-bearing status (immediate and in the ED)	1
Explains to patient:	
• No evidence of significant injury	1
• Analgesia advice	1
• Mobilization advice	1
• Return to sport advice	1
• Written info sheet	1
• Appropriate safety net	1
Demonstrates systematic, organized approach	2
Global score from examiner	5
Global score from actor	5
Total	**35**

Question 58 Ultrasound

Instructions for candidate

This elderly man has been brought into the ED after complaining of severe abdominal pain. Please do a FAST examination to view his abdominal aorta, and to determine if there is any visible free fluid. Please tell the examiner your findings. The patient is haemodynamically stable and conscious.

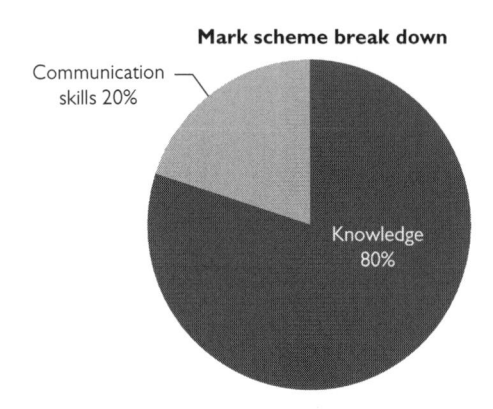

Mark scheme break down

- Communication skills 20%
- Knowledge 80%

Instructions for actor

You are an 86-year-old man. You were eating breakfast this morning and you suddenly got a severe pain in the centre of your tummy. Your wife called 999. You feel much better now you have been given some painkillers through a drip.

You have high BP and diabetes, but you can't remember the names of any of your medication. When the candidate uses the ultrasound, it doesn't cause you any discomfort.

Instructions for examiner

Please inform the candidate when they have 2 minutes left in the station. When they have 1 minute left, stop them, and ask them to present their findings.

Equipment required

Ultrasound machine
Ultrasound gel
Examination trolley

Curriculum mapping

Sections of the CEM (2010) curriculum relevant to this question include the following.

Common competencies

CC2 Clinical examination
CC4 Time management and decision-making
CC5 Decision-making and clinical reasoning
CC6 Patient as the central focus of care
CC12 Relationship with patients and communication

ACCS Acute presentations CT1&2

CAP1 Abdominal pain including loin pain
CAP2 Abdominal swelling, mass, and constipation

Question 58 Ultrasound

CAP3 Acute back pain
CAP23 Pain management

Mark scheme

Introduces self	1
Checks patient is comfortable	1
Explains purpose of scan:	
• To look at main blood vessel in abdomen	1
• To look for fluid in abdomen	1
• **Not** a detailed scan	1
Prepares patient:	
• Lies patient flat	1
• Exposes abdomen adequately	1
Prepares ultrasound scanner:	
• Enters patient details	1
• Correct type of scan set-up (abdominal)	1
• Correct probe selected	1
Warns patient about cold jelly	1
Demonstrates correct scan technique:	
• Familiar with depth, gain, focus settings	2
• Adequate orientation	1
• Systematic attempt overall	2
Takes aortic views:	
• Correct identification of aorta throughout length	1
• Attempted longitudinal views of proximal, middle, distal abdominal aorta	1
• Attempted transverse views of proximal, middle, distal abdominal aorta	1
• Correct use of measurement technique	1
• Correctly labelled	1
Examines for free fluid:	
• Hepatorenal pouch correctly identified	1
• Spleno-renal interface correctly identified	1
• Bladder correctly identified	1
• Pericardial space correctly identified	1
• Correctly labelled	1
Demonstrates familiarity with technique	2
Ensures patient dignity when scan finished	1
Explains results to patient	1
Explains additional tests needed	1
Global score from examiner	5
Global score from actor	5
Total	**40**

Question 59 Basic life support

Instructions for candidate

You are on the way to your night shift in the ED. You are walking across the hospital car park when you see a man collapsed on the ground. He is not moving. Please assess him and give him any treatment you can.

Mark scheme break down

Knowledge 100%

Instructions for examiner

The candidate should undertake 'out of hospital, single rescuer, adult basic life support' on this patient. The patient (manikin) is unresponsive, is not breathing, and has no palpable pulse or signs of life. He feels cold and has fixed dilated pupils. There are no changes despite the candidate's efforts to resuscitate him.

If asked the following questions by the candidate, you may give the following information:

There is no mobile phone reception in the car park
The nearest telephone is 5 minutes by foot, inside the hospital building
The car park is not covered by the 'crash' team (hospital cardiac arrest team)
There are no passers-by

Equipment required

Basic manikin
Cleaning wipes

Curriculum mapping

Sections of the CEM (2010) curriculum relevant to this question include the following.

Common competencies

CC4 Time management and decision-making
CC6 Patient as the central focus of care
CC15 Communication with colleagues and cooperation

ACCS Major presentations CT1&2

CMP2 Cardiorespiratory arrest

Guidelines available

http://www.resus.org.uk/pages/blsalgo.pdf

Question 59 Basic life support

Mark scheme

Checks safe to approach	1
Checks for response, e.g. 'Are you ok?'	1
Shouts for help	1
Opens airway	1
Adequately checks breathing for maximum 10 seconds	2
After establishing there is no breathing, attempts to call 999—this will involve leaving the patient—this must be done before starting CPR	1
Starts chest compressions	1
Uses correct technique for chest compressions—hands mid-point of chest with interlocking fingers, 5–6 cm depth of compression, rate 100–120	2
Delivers 2 rescue breaths	1
Uses correct technique for rescue breaths	2
Delivers 2 rescue breaths for 30 compressions or explains why they choose not to do mouth to mouth ventilation (infection risk)	1
Does not interrupt basic life support until another rescuer arrives or if signs of life/adequate breathing	1
Demonstrates systematic, organized approach	2
Global score from examiner	5
Global score from actor	5
Total	**27**

Question 60 Chest drain

Instructions for candidate
Your consultant has asked you to insert a right-sided chest drain in this patient who has a haemothorax. The patient has already been consented for the procedure by your consultant. Please demonstrate the correct technique for insertion of an intercostal chest drain.

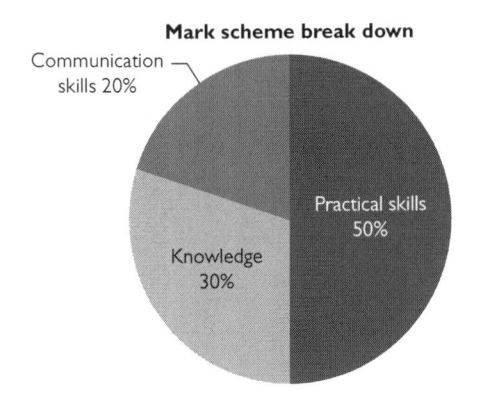

Mark scheme break down
- Communication skills 20%
- Knowledge 30%
- Practical skills 50%

Instructions for examiner
Observation only.

Please note, if it is not possible to obtain a 'model chest' for this station, the candidate could 'talk though' the procedure, using the equipment, in order to practise the station.

Equipment required
'Model' chest suitable for chest drain insertion
Appropriate X-ray
Chest drain insertion kit:

- Trolley
- Gloves
- Surgical gowns
- Surgical eye protectors/goggles
- Equipment for hand washing
- Sterile drapes
- Selection of chest drains of different sizes
- Local anaesthetic
- Underwater seal and connection tubing
- Needles and syringe
- Scalpel
- Blunt dissection instrument
- Sutures
- Needle holder
- Scissors
- Dressing
- Tape

Question 60 Chest drain

Curriculum mapping

Sections of the CEM (2010) curriculum relevant to this question include the following.

Common competencies

CC2 Clinical examination
CC3 Therapeutics and safe prescribing
CC5 Decision-making and clinical reasoning
CC6 Patient as the central focus of care
CC7 Prioritization of patient safety in clinical practice
CC10 Infection control
CC12 Relationship with patients and communication
CC15 Communication with colleagues and cooperation
CC18 Valid consent

ACCS Major presentations CT1&2

CMP3 Major trauma

ACCS Acute presentations CT1&2

CAP23 Pain management

Guidelines available

http://www.brit-thoracic.org.uk/portals/0/clinicalinformation/pleuraldisease/chestdrain-adults.pdf

Mark scheme

Introduces self	1
Explains diagnosis—haemothorax	1
Explains need for chest drain to remove blood and monitor further bleeding	1
Checks patient is comfortable/appropriate analgesia—IV opiates	1
Checks side of haemothorax, e.g. asks to see X-ray, confirms with patient	1
Checks patient understands procedure (patient has already been consented so is therefore aware of what is involved)	1
Prepares equipment adequately using sterile technique	2
Washes hands	1
Positions patient correctly (semireclined, right arm behind head—supported by helper)	1
Correctly identifies landmarks (5th intercostal space—anterior axillary line in triangle of safety—utilizing manubrio-sternal junction to identify 2nd rib)	2
Inserts local anaesthetic—correct choice and dose (1% plain lignocaine 3ml/kg to max 200 mg) and checks it has worked before starting	2
Makes appropriately sized skin incision with scalpel	1
Blunt dissects through muscle	1
Carries out finger sweep of pleura—does not lose track at any time	1
Inserts chest drain through incision	1
Connects drain to seal	1
Ensures chest drain is swinging and draining, noting initial amount of blood collected	1
Adequately secures drain with sutures and tape	1

Continued

Self-Assessment for the MCEM Part C

Continued

Applies dressing over drain	1
Communicates well with patient throughout	2
Indicates need for repeat CXR once procedure complete, is aware of indications for cardiothoracic referral	1
Global score from examiner	5
Global score from actor	5
Total	**35**

Question 61 Organ donation

Instructions for candidate

You are looking after a 24-year-old woman, Fiona, in the resuscitation room. She has been brought in after being hit by a motorbike when she was on a pedestrian crossing. Your consultant has discussed the patient with the regional neurosurgical centre. She has sustained a non-survivable head injury, which your consultant has already explained to her parents.

Your consultant is now dealing with another trauma call, but, since you have been involved in the case, has asked you to discuss potential organ donation with Fiona's family.

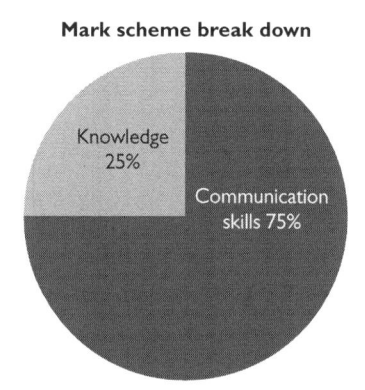

Mark scheme break down

Knowledge 25%
Communication skills 75%

Instructions for actor

You are the mother/father of a young woman called Fiona. She was a pedestrian who was knocked over by a motorcyclist earlier today. She was brought to hospital, where the team of doctors and nurses have been resuscitating her. They have done a CT scan which shows Fiona has severe bleeding and swelling on her brain. The consultant has explained this to you and shown you her CT scans. You have been told that there is no possibility Fiona can survive this type of injury, and there are no treatments or surgery that can help her. She is connected to a machine that is breathing for her and she is in a coma.

You know Fiona was on the organ donor register, because you remember having a conversation about it a couple of months ago. You think that Fiona would want to donate her organs, but you find the idea very upsetting. In particular, you can't bear the thought of anyone else having her eyes. You agree to speak to the organ donation team.

Instructions for examiner

Observation only.

Equipment required

None

Curriculum mapping

Sections of the CEM (2010) curriculum relevant to this question include the following.

Common competencies

CC12 Relationship with patients and communication
CC13 Breaking bad news
CC17 Ethics and confidentiality

Self-Assessment for the MCEM Part C

Mark scheme

Introduces self/ensures no pager/disturbances, etc.	1
Checks identity—Fiona's parents	1
Finds out what parents already know	1
Checks family understand diagnosis	2
Introduces subject of organ donation	1
Applies sensitive approach to discussion with family	2
Checks to see if Fiona is on organ donor register	1
Explains process of organ donation:	
• Led by organ donation team	1
• Further discussion with family	1
• Tests on patient to assess suitability	1
• Family can stipulate which organs are removed	1
• If organ donation is to go ahead, life support machines will be stopped, and family will be allowed to stay with the patient	1
• After death, once the family have said goodbye, the organs will be removed	1
• After donation, body will be returned to the family for the funeral	1
Gives opportunities for questions	1
Explains what will happen next—discussion with organ donation team	1
Global score from examiner	5
Global score from actor	5
Total	**28**

Question 62 Inhaler technique

Instructions for candidate

This is a 10-year-old patient called Jack who has been brought to the ED after having his first ever 'asthma attack'. He has a strong family history of asthma and a medical history of eczema and hay fever. He has previously had a few episodes of feeling wheezy over the last few years, which his mother has treated by giving him some puffs of her inhaler. He has never had his own inhaler.

Jack has been treated with a salbutamol inhaler via a spacer, and has been given some oral prednisolone. After a period of observation he is much improved, and you would like him to try salbutamol inhalers for the first time. Please teach Jack and his mother how to use his new inhaler and spacer.

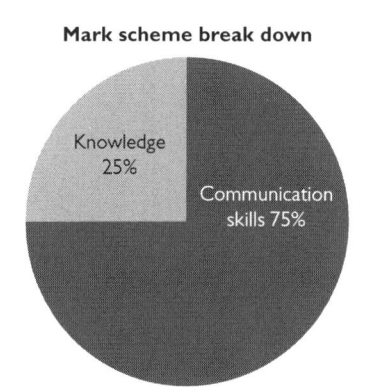

Mark scheme break down

- Knowledge 25%
- Communication skills 75%

Instructions for actors (child and parent)

You have used this inhaler for the first time today. You aren't sure how to use it by yourself, because the nurses have helped you so far. You are able to follow instructions given by the candidate.

Instructions for examiner

Observation only.

Equipment required

Selection of volumatics with mouth pieces and face masks
Salbutamol metered dose inhaler

Curriculum mapping

Sections of the CEM (2010) curriculum relevant to this question include the following.

Common competencies

CC3 Therapeutics and safe prescribing
CC6 Patient as the central focus of care
CC11 Management of long-term conditions and promoting patient self-care
CC12 Relationship with patients and communication
CC16 Health promotion and public health
CC23 Teaching and training

Paediatric acute presentations (PAPs)

PAP5 Breathing difficulties—recognize the critically ill and those who will need intubation and ventilation

Self-Assessment for the MCEM Part C

Guidelines available

http://www.brit-thoracic.org.uk/guidelines/asthma-guidelines.aspx

Mark scheme

Introduces self	1
Checks family understand diagnosis and plan	1
Explains treatment and how it works	1
Explains how often Jack needs to use inhalers when he goes home (10 puffs every 4–6 hours initially)	2
Describes asthma management plan + provides written plan	2
Describes technique:	
• Shake inhaler before use	1
• Selects correct size volumatic	1
• 10 breaths for each puff	1
• Normal breaths in and out with mouth around mouthpiece	1
Teaches how to look after volumatic—wash in soapy water, leave to drip dry	1
Allows Jack to try technique	1
Corrects Jack's technique	1
Invites questions	1
Revises asthma management plan, especially how to escalate use, when to seek help, and provides safety net by suggesting GP practice/asthma nurse follow-up	2
Global score from examiner	5
Global score from actor	5
Total	**27**

Question 63 Arterial line

Instructions for candidate
You have been asked to insert an arterial line in this patient who has had an out-of-hospital cardiac arrest and has been successfully resuscitated. Please insert the arterial line, obtain an arterial blood gas sample, and set up the pressure monitoring equipment.

Mark scheme break down

- Knowledge 50%
- Practical skills 50%

Instructions for examiner
Observation only.

Equipment required
Model for arterial line access
Cleaning solution
Sterile gloves, gown, and mask
Gauze swabs
Ultrasound machine
Local anaesthetic
Sterile saline
Selection of needles and syringes
Arterial catheters
Pressure bag
Fluid suitable for arterial line use
Giving set
Arterial line labels
Dressings
Arterial blood gas syringe

Curriculum mapping
Sections of the CEM (2010) curriculum relevant to this question include the following.

Common competencies
CC4 Time management and decision-making
CC7 Prioritization of patient safety in clinical practice
CC10 Infection control

Self-Assessment for the MCEM Part C

Mark scheme

Checks equipment	2
Sets up pressure bag, fluid, and giving set correctly	3
Sets up sterile tray with equipment	1
Examines patient to palpate radial/ulnar or femoral pulses	1
Washes hands and puts on sterile gloves	1
Cleans skin	1
Correctly inserts arterial line +/− ultrasound scan (USS) guidance	2
Secures arterial line	1
Takes sample in blood gas syringe for analysis	1
Connects fluid correctly	1
Flushes line safely	1
Zeros arterial line monitor	1
Obtains arterial line trace on monitor—checks against NIBP	1
Labels arterial line	1
Secures transducer in appropriate position	1
Demonstrates systematic, organized approach	2
Global score from examiner	5
Total	**26**

Question 64 Abdominal pain 1

Instructions for candidate

This patient has attended the ED with abdominal pain. He has a history of chronic abdominal pain, for which he has had many investigations. He has attended the ED six times in the last month with abdominal pain. On each occasion, he has been given analgesia, which has improved the pain, and he has been discharged home. His last set of blood tests were last week, which were all normal.

Today, one of the experienced ED nurses has asked you to talk to him. He has been assessed by one of your colleagues, who felt he had a soft abdomen and was concerned about drug-seeking behaviour. So they have refused to give him any more analgesia and asked him to leave. The patient is reluctant to go home because he is still in pain. Please talk to the patient to discuss his options.

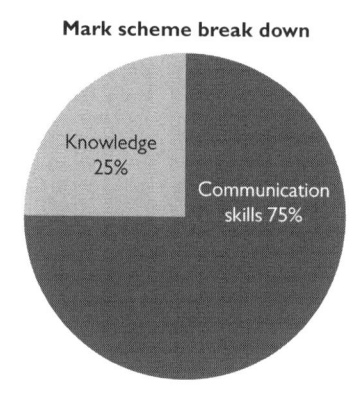

Mark scheme break down

- Knowledge 25%
- Communication skills 75%

Instructions for actor

You have been to the department today because you are feeling low and you wanted to get some strong painkillers like morphine to make you feel better. You are a recovering IV heroin user, who smokes cannabis occasionally but no longer uses anything else recreationally. You had an episode of abdominal pain several weeks ago, caused by gastroenteritis. The pain was very severe so one of your friends called an ambulance, who took you to the ED, where you were given IV morphine. Since then you have been back several times, even when the abdominal pain is not that bad.

You have noticed that the last couple of times you have gone to the hospital, the nurses and doctors seem reluctant to give you any morphine and suggest painkillers like paracetamol and ibuprofen. Today you have not been offered any painkillers, and the nurse has just told you that the doctor thinks you should go home. You are disappointed not to receive any morphine so you have asked to speak to a different doctor to see if they can prescribe you something stronger. You are willing to exaggerate your symptoms if they will give you some morphine. If they refuse to give you any morphine, you become aggressive and threaten to sue the hospital. If the doctor remains calm and challenges your drug-seeking behaviour, you tell them you will go to another hospital for a second opinion.

Instructions for examiner

Observation only.

Equipment required

None

Curriculum mapping

Sections of the CEM (2010) curriculum relevant to this question include the following.

Common competencies

CC1 History taking
CC3 Therapeutics and safe prescribing
CC11 Management of long-term conditions and promoting patient self-care
CC12 Relationship with patients and communication
CC15 Communication with colleagues and cooperation
CC16 Health promotion and public health
CC17 Ethics and confidentiality

ACCS Acute presentations CT1&2

CAP23 Pain management

Mark scheme

Introduces self	1
Checks patient's understanding of events so far	2
Summarizes patient's history	3
Uses open questions about reasons for attendance to ED	2
Discusses analgesic ladder	2
Explains why morphine is not offered as first analgesic	2
Refuses to prescribe morphine despite patient's protests	1
Does not antagonize patient, remains calm and professional and non-judgemental	2
Offers supportive options: GP, Drug and Alcohol Support Services	2
Global score from examiner	5
Global score from actor	5
Total	**27**

Question 65 Abdominal pain 2

Instructions for candidate
This 64-year-old man has attended the ED with abdominal pain. Please take a history and explain to the patient what you would like to do next.

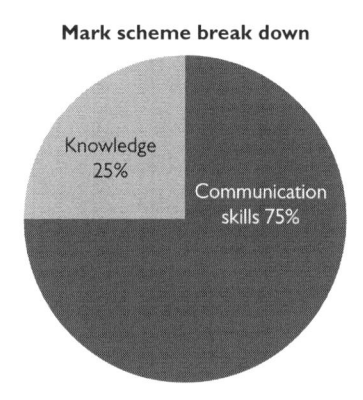

Mark scheme break down

- Knowledge 25%
- Communication skills 75%

Instructions for actor
You are a 64-year-old man who has had severe, sudden-onset abdominal pain about 2 hours ago. It happened when you were sat down watching television. It came on very suddenly, initially quite mild, then got much worse over a few minutes. It was in the centre of your tummy, radiating into the left flank. It made you feel dizzy and sick. You were given some morphine in the ambulance, on the way to hospital, about an hour ago, which made the pain go away. Now the pain is starting to come back. You still feel very dizzy and unwell.

You have not had any other symptoms. You have had no problems with passing urine or opening your bowels. You have not had any fevers. You have not eaten anything different from your wife, who is well. No other family members have abdominal pain. You are normally very fit and healthy. Yesterday you played a round of golf and felt fine. You have high BP and recently stopped smoking, having cut down from smoking 10 a day. You take a tablet for your BP and one for cholesterol, but you can't remember their names. You have no allergies.

Your father died of a heart attack aged 62, and your brother had a heart attack aged 65 but is still alive. You are a retired engineer. You are quite active, playing golf twice a week, and gardening. You can walk around the golf course without getting tired, but get out of breath quite quickly on walking uphill. You are anxious about what might have caused this abdominal pain, and are keen to get any investigations done as soon as possible. You ask the doctor what they think is the most likely diagnosis. If they give you a diagnosis, ask them about treatment and surgery.

Instructions for examiner
Observation only.
If the candidate asks, you can reassure them that the patient is haemodynamically stable.

Equipment required
None

Curriculum mapping
Sections of the CEM (2010) curriculum relevant to this question include the following.

Self-Assessment for the MCEM Part C

Common competencies

CC1 History taking
CC4 Time management and decision-making
CC5 Decision-making and clinical reasoning
CC6 Patient as the central focus of care
CC7 Prioritization of patient safety in clinical practice
CC8 Team work and patient safety
CC12 Relationship with patients and communication
CC13 Breaking bad news

ACCS Acute presentations CT1&2

CAP1 Abdominal pain including loin pain
CAP23 Pain management

Mark scheme

Introduces self	1
Checks patient is comfortable—asks if has had/requires analgesia	1
Uses combination open/closed questions to clarify points in history	1
Takes history of presenting complaint:	
• Description of abdominal pain	1
• Associated features	1
• Exacerbating/relieving factors	1
• Precipitating events	1
Takes past medical history	1
Asks about drug use	1
Asks about alcohol use	1
Asks about smoking history	1
Asks about family history	1
Explains:	
• Possible diagnosis is AAA	1
• Other diagnoses possible	1
• Further investigations include US scan and/or CT	1
• Needs to stay in hospital until this is ruled out	1
Invites questions	1
Explains treatment for leaking/ruptured aneurysm	1
Explains referral to vascular surgeons if required	1
Closure—reviews understanding with patient	1
Global score from examiner	5
Global score from actor	5
Total	**30**

Question 66 Hand examination

Instructions for candidate
This elderly lady has attended the ED with a 48-hour history of pain in her hands. Please examine her hands and describe your findings to the examiner.

Mark scheme break down
- Communication skills 20%
- Knowledge 80%

Instructions for actor
Allow the patient to examine you. Do not prompt them, e.g. by changing position. Please make it clear if they cause you any discomfort.

Instructions for examiner
Allow the candidate to examine the patient. One minute before the end, stop them and instruct them to describe their examination findings.

Equipment required
Pillow

Curriculum mapping
Sections of the CEM (2010) curriculum relevant to this question include the following.

Common competencies

CC2 Clinical examination
CC12 Relationship with patients and communication

ACCS Acute presentations CT1&2

CAP20 Limb pain and swelling—atraumatic
CAP23 Pain management

Mark scheme

Introduces self	1
Washes hands	1
Inspects general appearance	1
Inspects hands for deformities, swelling, colour change (palmer erythema), muscle wasting, scars, clubbing, nail pitting, etc.	2

Continued

Self-Assessment for the MCEM Part C

Continued

Exposure to the elbows (place on pillow)—look at elbows for rheumatoid nodules, psoriatic plaques	1
Palpates:	
• Warmth over joints	1
• Bony tenderness	1
• Thenar eminence	1
• Hypothenar eminence	1
• Feels along tendon sheaths, comments on thickening, trigger points, ganglions, etc.	1
Checks shumb movements (active and passive):	
• Abduction/adduction	1
• Flexion/extension	1
• Opposition	1
Checks finger movements (active and passive) including tendons:	
• Extension	1
• Flexion (deep and superficial)—specifically examines for flexor digitorum superficialis and profundus	1
Checks neurology:	
• Median nerve motor—'**LOAF**': **L**umbricals 1 & 2, **O**pponens pollicis, **A**bductor pollicis brevis, and **F**lexor pollicis brevis; sensory palmar side of thumb, index, middle, and half ring finger; nail bed of these fingers. Lateral part of palm is supplied by palmar cutaneous branch of median nerve	2
• Ulnar nerve motor—in the hand, via deep branch of ulnar nerve—'HOAF': **H**ypothenar muscles, **O**pponens digiti minimi, **A**bductor digiti minimi, **F**lexor digiti minimi; third and fourth lumbrical muscles; dorsal and palmar interossei; adductor pollicis; flexor pollicis brevis (deep head); palmaris brevis and sensory to fifth digit and medial half of fourth digit, and corresponding part of palm	2
• Radial nerve motor—in the hand: no motor innervation to intrinsic muscles. Forearm: innervates forearm muscles that provide extension of wrist, thumb, and all finger MCPJs and sensory dorsal aspect of radial two-thirds of hand and thumb; dorsal aspect of thumb, index, middle, and radial half of ring finger to proximal interphalangeal (PIP) joint	2
Therefore movements that should be assessed are: wrist flexion, wrist extension, finger extension, finger flexion, finger abduction, thumb abduction, thumb opposition	
Carries out vascular check:	
• Radial and ulnar pulses	1
• CRT	1
Carries out functional assessment e.g. writing, doing up a button, power grip, pincer grip, fine grip (picking up a small object)	1
Displays systematic, organized approach	1
Concisely summarizes findings	3
Thanks patient	1
Global score from examiner	5
Global score from actor	5
Total	**41**

Question 67 Abdominal examination

Instructions for candidate
This 7-year-old boy has attended the ED with a 24-hour history of abdominal pain which has now settled. Please examine his abdomen and describe your findings to the examiner.

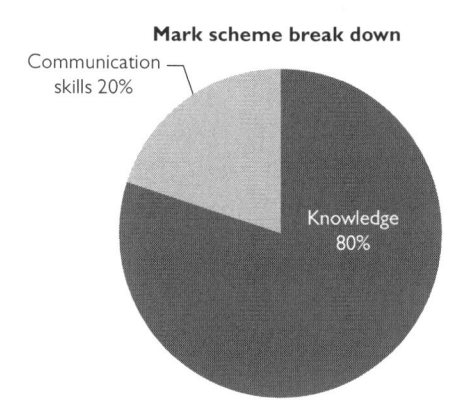

Mark scheme break down
- Communication skills 20%
- Knowledge 80%

Instructions for actor
Allow the patient to examine you. You have mild tenderness in the centre of your abdomen. Do not prompt them, e.g. by changing position. Please make it clear if they cause you any discomfort.

Instructions for examiner
Allow the candidate to examine the patient. One minute before the end, stop them and instruct them to describe their examination findings. Do not prompt the candidate.

Equipment required
None

Curriculum mapping
Sections of the CEM (2010) curriculum relevant to this question include the following.

Common competencies
CC2 Clinical examination
CC12 Relationship with patients and communication

Paediatric acute presentations (PAPs)
PAP1 Abdominal pain
PAP15 Pain in children

Self-Assessment for the MCEM Part C

Mark scheme

Introduces self	1
Washes hands	1
Explains need for examination	1
Offers chaperone	1
Checks for analgesia requirement	1
Ensures patient sitting at 45 degrees	1
Inspects: general appearance, hands (clubbing, palmar erythema, etc.), face: eyes for jaundice (icterus, xanthelasmata), mouth for anaemia, telangiectasia, pigmentation, ulcers, as well as any clues/props placed near patient	2
Lies patient flat and adequately exposes patient (from nipples to knees)—while maintaining modesty	1
Inspects abdomen for distension, bruising, masses from end of the bed	2
Palpates: demonstrates organized, systematic approach utilizing quadrants of abdomen:	
• Light superficial palpation	1
• Deeper palpation	1
• Specifically feels for AAA	1
• Liver	1
• Spleen	1
• Kidneys	1
• Shifting dullness for ascites	1
Ballots kidneys	1
Percusses liver, any organomegaly or distension	1
Auscultates for bowel sounds + for renal bruits	1
Inspects and palpates groins, comments on femoral pulses and lymph nodes	1
States to complete examination would also need to inspect and palpate external genitalia	1
States to complete examination would also need to do rectal examination	1
Requests baseline clinical observations + urine dipstick test	1
Demonstrates systematic, organized approach	1
Concisely summarizes findings	2
Thanks patient	1
Global score from examiner	5
Global score from actor	5
Total	**39**

Question 68 Lumbar puncture

Instructions for candidate

This patient is being investigated for a subarachnoid haemorrhage. They attended the ED yesterday with a severe headache, the CT head scan was reported as showing no abnormalities, and 12 hours have passed since the onset.

The patient has already been consented for the procedure by your consultant and has no contraindications for LP. Please demonstrate an appropriate technique for performing an LP.

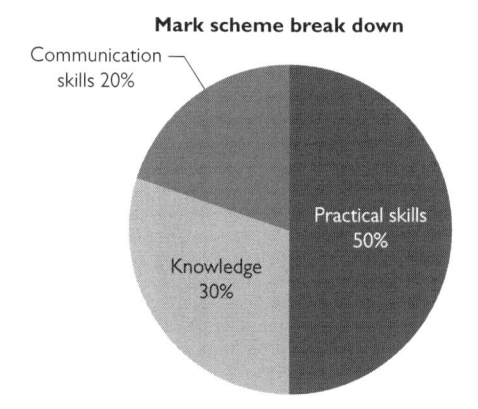

Mark scheme break down

- Communication skills 20%
- Knowledge 30%
- Practical skills 50%

Instructions for examiner

Observation only.

Please note, if it is not possible to obtain a 'model' for this station, the candidate could 'talk through' the procedure, using the equipment, in order to practise the station.

Equipment required

'Model' suitable for LP
Maybe normal CT head scan
LP kit:

- Trolley
- Gloves
- Surgical gowns
- Surgical eye protectors/goggles
- Equipment for hand washing
- Sterile drapes
- Selection of spinal needles of different sizes
- Local anaesthetic
- Manometer
- Collection bottles (three universal containers plus biochemistry tubes)
- Cleaning solution
- Dressing

Curriculum mapping

Sections of the CEM (2010) curriculum relevant to this question include the following.

Self-Assessment for the MCEM Part C

Common competencies

CC2 Clinical examination
CC6 Patient as the central focus of care
CC10 Infection control
CC12 Relationship with patients and communication
CC18 Valid consent

ACCS Acute presentations CT1&2

CAP17 Headache
CAP23 Pain management

Mark scheme

Introduces self	1
Explains procedure or checks patient understands procedure, discusses potential side-effects/complications—especially post-procedural headache	2
Explains why LP needed. Is aware of other options should candidate not be successful, e.g. fluoroscopic guidance, MRI	2
Checks patient is comfortable	1
Checks equipment	1
Positions patient adequately—lateral (fetal) or supine position	1
Prepares equipment adequately using sterile technique—chooses a pencil-point needle with introducer (as decreases risk of LP-associated headache as the point spits fibres rather than cuts fibres). Correctly constructs manometer	2
Washes hands	1
Correctly identifies landmarks (anterior superior iliac spine—correlates to L3/4 position)	1
Inserts local anaesthetic (plain lignocaine 3 mg/kg) and checks it has worked before starting	1
Inserts spinal needle using correct technique	1
Obtains cerebrospinal fluid (CSF)	1
Correctly measures opening pressure value	1
Correctly collects samples in appropriately numbered containers	1
Removes needle and covers with dressing	1
Advises patient about post LP care	1
Clears away sharps	1
Clarifies what tests will be requested—cell count, microscopy, culture, and sensitivities (MCS), xanthochromia, glucose, protein	2
Labels sample bottles—requests envelope so that xanthochromia specimen can be transported avoiding exposure to daylight	1
Communicates well with patient throughout	2
Global score from examiner	5
Global score from actor	5
Total	**35**

Question 69 Hypothermia

Instructions for candidate

You are called to resus to see a 40-year-old man who has been pulled out of a lake after falling in whilst walking his dog. You have an experienced nurse and a healthcare assistant from the ED with you. Please assess the patient and treat as necessary.

Mark scheme break down

- Team leadership skills 50%
- Knowledge 50%

Instructions for examiner

You may provide the candidate with the following information if requested:

A—airway clear
B—patient is apnoeic, no recordable SaO_2
C—no palpable pulse, very cold centrally and peripherally, no recordable BP
D—temperature 28°C

Monitoring shows ventricular fibrillation (VF). After one shock, this changes to PEA at a rate of 10–15. There are no external signs of injury visible. If active warming measures are commenced, temperature starts to increase slowly but patient remains in cardiac arrest until the end of the station.

Equipment required

Standard adult resuscitation equipment (see introductory section)

Curriculum mapping

Sections of the CEM (2010) curriculum relevant to this question include the following.

Common competencies

CC1 History taking
CC2 Clinical examination
CC3 Therapeutics and safe prescribing
CC4 Time management and decision-making
CC5 Decision-making and clinical reasoning
CC8 Team work and patient safety
CC15 Communication with colleagues and cooperation

Self-Assessment for the MCEM Part C

ACCS Major presentations CT1&2

CMP2 Cardiorespiratory arrest

Guidelines available

http://www.resus.org.uk/pages/alsalgo.pdf

Mark scheme

Gives oxygen	1
Applies A B C D E approach	2
Gives prompt CPR	1
Delivers shocks promptly, appropriately, and safely—recognizes that shocks may be ineffective until temperature returns to above 30°C	1
Calls for senior EM/anaesthetic/ITU assistance	1
Considers '4 Hs' and '4 Ts'	1
Intubates properly	1
Promptly diagnoses VF cardiac arrest	1
Gains IV/intraosseus (IO) access, blood test taken + VBG (+ measures blood glucose)	1
Checks temperature	1
Requests active rewarming measures	1
Ensures wet clothing removed, patient dried	2
Gives adrenaline appropriately—recognizes need to stop/withhold drugs until temperature above 30°C	1
Repeats temperature, ensures active warming commenced, gives humidified oxygen, gives warmed fluids, considers bladder lavage, etc.	1
Considers relatives	1
Displays team leadership skills	2
Global score from examiner	5
Total	**24**

Question 70 Infant resuscitation

Instructions for candidate

You are the ED registrar on nights in a busy district general hospital. Ambulance control has just phoned to say they have a 1-week-old baby in cardiac arrest coming to you by ambulance. They are 2 minutes away. Basic life support is in progress.

You have one paediatric nurse and one ED nurse with you. You may use the first minute of this station to make any calculations you think you might need.

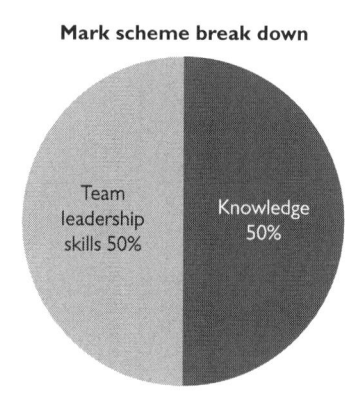

Mark scheme break down

- Team leadership skills 50%
- Knowledge 50%

Instructions for actor

You are a staff nurse in the ED. You know where all the equipment is kept and can hand it to the candidate, but you don't act without being clearly instructed to do so.

Instructions for examiner

If asked by the candidate, give the following information:

The baby was found unresponsive in his cot this morning when his mother went to check on him. She had put him to sleep 4 hours earlier. The baby looks full term from his size. His estimated weight is 4 kg.
The ambulance crew have been doing basic life support for 25 minutes already.

On initial assessment:

A—clear
B—apnoeic
C—no pulse or signs of life, asystole on monitor
D—fixed dilated pupils, blood glucose 6.2, temperature 35.4°C

No rashes or bruises. There is no response to basic airway manoeuvres, ventilation, CPR, or other treatment. You may ask the candidate what they would like to do next, but do not prompt.

In order for the station to progress, you will need to artificially speed up the scenario, e.g. by allowing 2-minute intervals to pass quickly. By the end of the scenario, if the candidate has not already started to consider stopping resuscitation, ask the candidate what they are thinking at this stage, as a prompt.

Equipment required

Standard paediatric resuscitation equipment (see introductory section)

Curriculum mapping

Sections of the CEM (2010) curriculum relevant to this question include the following.

Common competencies

CC1 History taking
CC2 Clinical examination
CC3 Therapeutics and safe prescribing
CC4 Time management and decision-making
CC5 Decision-making and clinical reasoning
CC6 Patient as the central focus of care
CC8 Team work and patient safety
CC12 Relationship with patients and communication
CC15 Communication with colleagues and cooperation

Paediatric major presentations (PMPs)

PMP3 Cardiorespiratory arrest

Guidelines available

http://www.resus.org.uk/pages/palsalgo.pdf

Mark scheme

Calls for paediatric resuscitation team	1
Prepares calculations correctly	2
Quickly takes handover from ambulance crew	2
Stops resuscitation to reassess	1
Checks and clears airway	1
Places head in neutral position	1
Looks, listens, and feels for respiratory effort for 10 seconds	1
Gives 5 adequate rescue breaths	1
Checks for signs of life and palpable pulse	1
Starts CPR (ratio of breaths to compressions 15:2)	1
Carries out adequate CPR technique (or corrects colleagues)	1
Connects cardiac monitor/paddles	1
Starts timing for 2-minute intervals	1
Attempts IV/IO access	1
Gives adrenaline at correct dose according to weight	1
Mentions/undertakes intubation	1
Checks blood glucose	1
Considers/gives fluid bolus	1
Reassesses and recognizes no response to resuscitation—considers stopping resuscitation	1
Considers/involves parents in discussions about stopping resuscitation	1
Displays team leadership skills	2
Global score from examiner	5
Total	**29**

Question 71 Seizure 2

Instructions for candidate
This 17-year-old patient has attended the ED because she has had a seizure in the street. She is known to have epilepsy and does not come to hospital each time she has a fit, but a passer-by called 999 today. You notice that the girl has been brought to hospital several times in the last few months with seizures. Please explore the reasons for her increased seizure frequency.

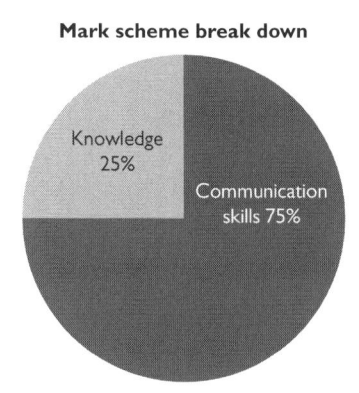

Mark scheme break down

- Knowledge 25%
- Communication skills 75%

Instructions for actor
You are a 17-year-old girl who has had epilepsy for the last 8 years. You are prescribed a medication called 'epilim' which you are supposed to take every day. You have stopped taking your tablets because you have read the leaflet that comes with the tablets, and it said the tablets can cause weight gain. You have not talked to anyone about this. Your mother took you to the GP to find out why you were having more seizures than normal, and the GP mentioned that sometimes teenagers find they have seizures more often than normal for no obvious reason. Your GP has referred you back to the neurologist at the hospital, but you haven't had an appointment yet.

A 'typical' seizure for you means that you feel 'funny' for about 5 minutes, and then you fall to the floor. Your arms and legs shake for about 5 minutes and you are not aware of anything around you. When you stop shaking, you gradually wake up but feel really tired for about an hour afterwards. If this happens at home, your parents stay with you until you are back to normal, and you only come to hospital if someone calls an ambulance.

When you take your medication properly, you only have a seizure once a year or so. At the moment, you are having seizures every 3 or 4 weeks. They mostly happen in the evenings when you are at home, feeling tired after a busy day at college. You have had two seizures outside in the street when you've been out shopping, which you found really embarrassing.

You have no other medical problems. You take no other medication and have no allergies. You are a college student, studying A levels. You have a big group of friends. You live with your parents and two younger brothers. You get on reasonably well with your family. You don't smoke. You drink alcohol at weekends with your friends when you go out, but don't like getting drunk in case it causes a seizure. You occasionally smoke cannabis when friends bring it to parties, but don't take any other drugs.

If the doctor asks about why you think you are having more seizures, you should tell them that you're not taking your medication and the reason why. If they make suggestions about your epilepsy, you agree to these.

Instructions for examiner
Observation only.

Equipment required
None

Curriculum mapping
Sections of the CEM (2010) curriculum relevant to this question include the following.

Common competencies
CC1 History taking
CC6 Patient as the central focus of care
CC7 Prioritization of patient safety in clinical practice
CC11 Management of long-term conditions and promoting patient self-care
CC12 Relationship with patients and communication
CC16 Health promotion and public health

ACCS Acute presentations CT1&2
CAP15 Fits/seizure

Mark scheme

Introduces self	1
Takes history of presenting complaint—seizures	2
Explores change in seizure frequency:	
• Current frequency	1
• Previous frequency	1
• Type of seizures	1
• Medication	1
• Stress/drugs/alcohol	1
• Sleep patterns	1
• Recent illnesses	1
Explores medication compliance	2
Asks about past medical history	1
Asks about medications and allergies	2
Asks about social history	1
Investigates reasons for poor medication compliance	1
Explores understanding of medications	2
Makes suggestions/reassurances about medication	2
Recommends neurology/epilepsy nurse follow-up	1
Invites questions	1
Conducts consultation in non-judgemental way	2
Global score from examiner	5
Global score from actor	5
Total	**35**

Question 72 Burns

Instructions for candidate

You are on duty in a large district general hospital. An ambulance is en route to you from half a mile away with a 60-year-old man from a garage fire. He has a reduced level of consciousness and is tachycardic. You have an ED nurse with you.

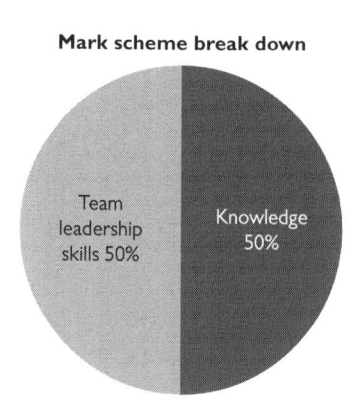

Mark scheme break down

- Team leadership skills 50%
- Knowledge 50%

Instructions for actor

You are a staff nurse in the ED. You know where all the equipment is kept and can hand it to the candidate, but you don't act without being clearly instructed to do so.

Instructions for examiner

When asked by the candidate, you may provide the following information:

A—burns visible to face and lips, swollen lips, carbonaceous sputum in mouth, noisy breathing improves with suction, will tolerate airway adjuncts

B—RR 18, saturations 90% on air, improved once oxygen given, burns to entire anterior chest, reasonable air entry throughout

C—pulse = 120, BP 90/70, CRT = 3 seconds. No IV access

D—E2, M3, V2

E—blood glucose = 6

Mixture of full and partial thickness burns to face, neck, anterior chest, abdomen, and both legs. Posterior surface of body not burned

Approximate weight 100 kg

Approximate 40% burns

Equipment required

Standard adult resuscitation equipment (see introductory section)
Manikin made up with burns as described

Curriculum mapping

Sections of the CEM (2010) curriculum relevant to this question include the following.

Self-Assessment for the MCEM Part C

Common competencies

CC1 History taking
CC2 Clinical examination
CC3 Therapeutics and safe prescribing
CC4 Time management and decision-making
CC5 Decision-making and clinical reasoning
CC6 Patient as the central focus of care
CC7 Prioritization of patient safety in clinical practice
CC8 Team work and patient safety
CC10 Infection control
CC15 Communication with colleagues and cooperation

ACCS Major presentations CT1&2

CMP3 Major trauma

ACCS Acute presentations CT1&2

CAP35 Ventilatory support

Mark scheme

Calls for trauma team (senior help and anaesthetist)	1
Ensures c-spine immobilization throughout	2
Gives prompt oxygen	1
Provides suction of airway and simple airway manoeuvres	1
Decides early intubation is a priority by an experienced practitioner	1
Carries out sequential A B C D E assessment	2
Assesses percentage burn	1
Assesses breathing—respiration rate, SaO_2, work of breathing	1
Appreciates that burns may restrict ventilation, considers need for escharotomies	1
Obtains IV/IO access	1
Takes bloods including blood glucose	1
Obtains arterial blood gas sample for carbon monoxide and cyanide poisoning	1
Gives IV fluid bolus	2
Reassesses after fluid bolus	1
Assesses cause of hypovolaemia and recognizes early hypovolaemia likely to be due to trauma, and delayed hypovolaemia due to burns	1
Considers Parkland fluid formula	1
Assesses level of consciousness prior to anaesthesia	1
Covers burns with appropriate dressing	1
Considers analgesia	1
Considers/demonstrates communication with burns team	1
Considers tetanus	1
Considers trauma imaging	1
Displays team leadership skills	2
Global score from examiner	5
Total	**32**

Question 73 Anaphylaxis

Instructions for candidate

You are called to resus to see a 20-year-old man who is having an allergic reaction after eating some nuts. You have an experienced nurse from the ED with you. Please assess the patient and treat as necessary.

Mark scheme break down

- Team leadership skills 50%
- Knowledge 50%

Instructions for actor

You are a staff nurse in the ED. You know where all the equipment is kept and can hand it to the candidate, but you don't act without being clearly instructed to do so.

Instructions for examiner

You may provide the candidate with the following information if requested:

A—stridor, swollen lips
B—audible wheeze, reasonable air entry, SaO_2 85% on air, 92% on 15 L oxygen, RR 25
C—HR 120, BP 90/70, peripherally vasodilated, CRT 3 seconds
D—GCS 15, very anxious
Urticarial rash to face and neck

The patient continues to deteriorate until the candidate gives IM adrenaline (regardless of other treatment given). Once adrenaline has been given, the patient slowly starts to improve. If the candidate requests that they want to intubate the patient, advise them that the equipment is being made ready and the anaesthetist will do this for them.

Equipment required

Standard adult resuscitation equipment (see introductory section)

Curriculum mapping

Sections of the CEM (2010) curriculum relevant to this question include the following.

Common competencies

CC1 History taking
CC2 Clinical examination
CC3 Therapeutics and safe prescribing
CC4 Time management and decision-making

CC5 Decision-making and clinical reasoning
CC6 Patient as the central focus of care
CC7 Prioritization of patient safety in clinical practice
CC8 Team work and patient safety
CC15 Communication with colleagues and cooperation

ACCS Major presentations CT1&2

CMP1 Anaphylaxis

Guidelines available

http://www.resus.org.uk/pages/reaction.pdf

Mark scheme

Introduces self to patient	1
Follows A B C D E approach	2
Calls for senior EM/anaesthetic/ITU assistance early	1
Assesses airway	2
Recognizes potential difficult airway, calls for help, and prepares for intubation	2
Gives IM adrenaline **before** moving on	2
Assesses breathing	2
Gives salbutamol nebulizer (and IM adrenaline if not already given)	1
Assesses circulation	1
Considers lying patient flat, to elevate legs (or specifically declines to do this, e.g. if concerned about the effect this might have on the patient's airway)	2
Obtains IV access	1
Gives the following:	
• IV fluid bolus	1
• IV hydrocortisone	1
• IV chlorphenamine	1
Reassesses patient	2
Describes ongoing management plan that includes:	
• Admission for a period of observation to detect biphasic reactions	1
• Allergy testing in clinic	1
• Prescription of EpiPen® to take home when fit for discharge	1
Demonstrates adequate team leadership skills	2
Global score from examiner	5
Total	**32**

Question 74 Antibiotic requesting

Instructions for candidate
You have been asked to speak to the mother of a 4-year-old patient (Georgia) who attended the ED with a sore throat. You have taken a history and diagnosed a viral upper respiratory tract infection. Please advise the parents before discharging Georgia.

Mark scheme break down

- Knowledge 25%
- Communication skills 75%

Instructions for actor
You are the mother of a 4-year-old, Georgia. You would like some antibiotics for Georgia as you think she has tonsillitis. She has had this several times before, and if she doesn't have antibiotics it takes a week to go away, whereas it clears up in a couple of days of starting antibiotics. Your GP has referred Georgia to the ear, nose, throat (ENT) specialist because she has had so many infections.

You normally go to your GP about this sort of thing, but there are no appointments for a couple of days, and you came to the ED to get hold of some antibiotics so they would start working straight away. If the doctor gives you a prescription for antibiotics, you are very grateful and leave quickly to collect your prescription. If the doctor is reluctant to give you a prescription, you should try to persuade them that antibiotics are the only things that make a difference.

Instructions for examiner
Observation only.

Equipment required
None

Curriculum mapping
Sections of the CEM (2010) curriculum relevant to this question include the following.

Common competencies

CC5 Decision-making and clinical reasoning
CC6 Patient as the central focus of care
CC11 Management of long-term conditions and promoting patient self-care
CC12 Relationship with patients and communication
CC14 Complaints and medical error

Self-Assessment for the MCEM Part C

Paediatric acute presentations (PAPs)

PAP8 ENT
PAP9 Fever in all age groups
PAP15 Pain in children

Mark scheme

Introduces self	1
Confirms Georgia's mother's identity	2
Explains diagnosis of viral upper respiratory tract infection	2
Explains treatment consists of analgesia, observation and **not** antibiotics	3
Answers mother's questions about antibiotics	2
Explains why antibiotics are not recommended:	
• Mentions National Institute for Health and Care Excellence (NICE) guidelines	1
• Offers patient information sheet	1
Deals adequately with concerns	3
Remains professional and polite when challenged	2
Invites questions	1
Safety netting—provides advice, including when to return to the ED	1
Shows non-verbal communication skills	2
Global score from examiner	5
Global score from actor	5
Total	**31**

Question 75 Pelvic examination

Instructions for candidate
This 65-year-old woman has attended the ED complaining of pelvic pain for the last 2 months. She thinks she can feel a lump in her right lower abdomen. She has not been to her GP but this week is staying with her daughter who has brought her along to get it sorted out once and for all. Please do a pelvic examination on this patient (using the model) and explain your findings to the patient, including any investigations you would recommend.

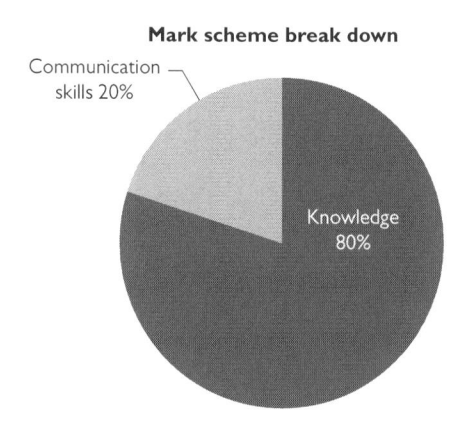

Mark scheme break down

- Communication skills 20%
- Knowledge 80%

Instructions for actor
You are very anxious about the pain and lump in your pelvis. You are worried it may be cancer. You agree to an examination (this will be done on the model pelvis). When the candidate is examining the model pelvis, please indicate that it is painful when the right lower abdomen is palpated. When the candidate explains the diagnosis, you should ask 'Is this cancer?' You agree to any investigations that the candidate suggests.

Instructions for examiner
Observation only.

If there is a pelvic model available, it should be set up to simulate a mass in the right iliac fossa. If no such model is available, the candidate could 'talk through' the process of bimanual and speculum examination. If the candidate does not explain their findings to the patient, interrupt them 1 minute before the end of the station and ask them to do so.

Equipment required
Actor
Pelvic model for bimanual and speculum examination
Gloves
Speculum
Lubrication
Screens for privacy
Sheet to cover patient
Gown

Curriculum mapping

Sections of the CEM (2010) curriculum relevant to this question include the following.

Common competencies

CC2 Clinical examination
CC5 Decision-making and clinical reasoning
CC6 Patient as the central focus of care
CC12 Relationship with patients and communication
CC17 Ethics and confidentiality
CC18 Valid consent

ACCS Acute presentations CT1&2

CAP26 Pelvic pain

Mark scheme

Introduces self	1
Offers analgesia or checks if analgesia already prescribed	1
Explains need for examination	2
Explains details of examination	2
Obtains verbal consent for examination	2
Offers chaperone	1
Ensures privacy	1
Allows patient to undress in private	1
Carries out bimanual examination	2
Checks temperature of Cusco speculum before use	1
Appropriately uses Cusco speculum	2
Allows patient to get dressed	1
Explains findings	2
Explains investigations needed, including ultrasound scan and blood tests	2
Invites questions	1
Demonstrates systematic, organized approach	2
Global score from examiner	5
Global score from actor	5
Total	**34**

Question 76 Seizure 3

Instructions for candidate

An ambulance is on the way to you with a 3-year-old who has been fitting for 15 minutes. They are 5 minutes away. They have been unable to get any IV access but have given the child rectal diazepam. Please assess the child. You have one paediatric nurse and one ED nurse with you. You may use the first minute of this station to make any calculations you think you might need.

Mark scheme break down

- Team leadership skills 50%
- Knowledge 50%

Instructions for actor

You are a staff nurse in the ED. You know where all the equipment is kept and can hand it to the candidate, but you don't act without being clearly instructed to do so.

Instructions for examiner

If asked by the candidate, give the following information. The child was found fitting in his cot by his mother today. She had put him to sleep an hour earlier. His mother told the ambulance crew that he has had diarrhoea and vomiting for the last 2 days and has been having fevers on and off, and has not had anything to eat or drink all day today.

On initial assessment:

Visible tonic clonic movements

A—airway occluded with secretions, improves with suctioning but still noisy. Unable to insert oropharyngeal airway due to trismus. Noisy breathing improves with insertion of nasopharyngeal airway

B—saturations 80%, blue lips, RR 30, reasonable air entry throughout, no focal signs

C—HR 150, CRT 3 seconds

BM 2.4

Temperature 39.2°C

No rashes

You may ask the candidate what they would like to do next, but do not prompt. In order for the station to progress, you will need to artificially speed up the scenario, e.g. by allowing intervals between drug treatments to pass quickly.

Equipment required

Standard paediatric resuscitation equipment (see introductory section)
White board and pen for weight/dose calculations

Self-Assessment for the MCEM Part C

Curriculum mapping

Sections of the CEM (2010) curriculum relevant to this question include the following.

Common competencies

CC1 History taking
CC2 Clinical examination
CC3 Therapeutics and safe prescribing
CC4 Time management and decision-making
CC5 Decision-making and clinical reasoning
CC6 Patient as the central focus of care
CC7 Prioritization of patient safety in clinical practice
CC8 Team work and patient safety
CC12 Relationship with patients and communication
CC15 Communication with colleagues and cooperation

Paediatric major presentations (PMPs)

PMP6 Unconscious child

Paediatric acute presentations (PAPs)

PAP9 Fever in all age groups

Mark scheme

Calls for paediatric resuscitation team	1
Prepares calculations correctly	2
Quickly takes handover from ambulance crew	2
Follows structured A B C D E approach	2
Checks and clears airway with suction	1
Uses airway adjunct	1
Looks, listens, and feels for respiratory effort for 10 seconds	1
Gives oxygen via non-rebreather mask	1
Checks for signs of life and palpable pulse	1
Checks blood glucose	1
Attempts IV/IO access and takes blood for hypoglycaemia screening tests	1
Gives IV dextrose in response to hypoglycaemia (2 ml/kg of 10% dextrose)	1
Checks temperature	1
Checks pupils	1
Gives benzodiazepine at correct dose according to weight	1
Is aware of timing until next drug	1
Gives phenytoin at correct dose	1
Considers/gives IV antibiotics	1
Considers/gives paracetamol	1
Considers/discusses rapid sequence induction of anaesthesia and calls appropriate help	1
Displays effective team leadership	2
Global score from examiner	5
Total	**30**

Question 77 Vaginal bleeding

Instructions for candidate

This 34-year-old woman who is 16 weeks pregnant has come to the ED with vaginal bleeding and pelvic pain. Since being in the department she has passed a large amount of products into a towel, including some recognizable foetal matter.

She is haemodynamically stable. Please explain to her that you would like to examine her, and explain what will happen next.

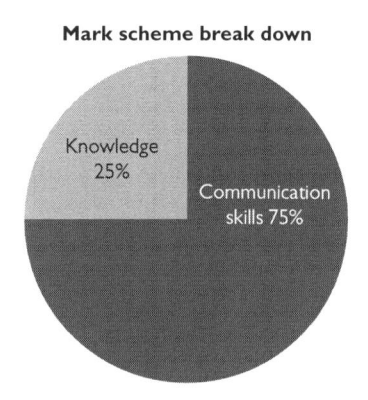

Mark scheme break down

- Knowledge 25%
- Communication skills 75%

Instructions for actor

You are a 34-year-old woman who is 16 weeks pregnant. This is your first pregnancy. You conceived after three cycles of in vitro fertilization (IVF). You are having fertility treatment for unexplained infertility. Your partner is currently away on a business trip in Singapore. You woke up this morning with some dull pain in your lower abdomen. About an hour ago, you started bleeding. You have passed a lot of blood and some 'lumps' and clots into a sanitary towel. You phoned your midwife who told you to come to the ED.

You have been given some painkillers by the nurse and the pain is much better, but you are terrified you have had a miscarriage. It has taken you 5 years to get pregnant and everything seemed to be going fine so far. You have no medical problems.

Instructions for examiner

Observation only.

Equipment required

None

Curriculum mapping

Sections of the CEM (2010) curriculum relevant to this question include the following.

Common competencies

CC1 History taking
CC5 Decision-making and clinical reasoning
CC6 Patient as the central focus of care
CC10 Infection control
CC12 Relationship with patients and communication
CC13 Breaking bad news

Self-Assessment for the MCEM Part C

ACCS Acute presentations CT1&2
CAP34 Vaginal bleeding

Mark scheme

Introduces self	1
Checks correct identity	1
Checks to see if next of kin/friend available	1
Establishes what is already known	2
Explains diagnosis is probable miscarriage	2
Offers sympathy	1
Explains need to do speculum to remove tissue in cervical os	2
Explains will be referred to gynaecology	1
Explains will have ultrasound scan to confirm diagnosis and determine if any retained products	1
Explains may need operation if there are retained products	1
Invites questions	1
Answers questions adequately	2
Global score from examiner	5
Global score from actor	5
Total	**26**

Question 78 Febrile convulsion

Instructions for candidate
You have been asked to speak to the mother of a 4-year-old patient (Adam) who was brought into the ED by ambulance after having a seizure at home. You have taken a history and diagnosed a febrile convulsion secondary to a viral upper respiratory tract infection. Adam has had a period of observation in your paediatric clinical decision unit. Please advise the parents before discharging Adam.

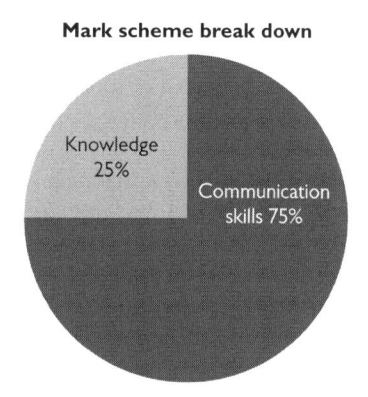

Mark scheme break down

- Knowledge 25%
- Communication skills 75%

Instructions for actor
You are the mother of a 4-year-old, Adam, who was taken to hospital earlier today after having a seizure. He has had a cold for a couple of days and you have been giving him regular Calpol® for his fevers. You put him in bed for a nap today because he looked tired, and after a few minutes you heard him shaking. You found him in bed having a seizure. He has never done this before, so you called 999. He stopped fitting just as the ambulance pulled up at the house. The ambulance crew told you his temperature was 39.5°C and gave him some ibuprofen.

He has been observed for a few hours and seems almost back to his normal self. The nurses have told you that Adam will probably be discharged home shortly. You are terrified that this might happen again. If the diagnosis is explained thoroughly to you, you are happy to take Adam home. If not, you refuse to leave and ask to stay in hospital overnight.

Instructions for examiner
Observation only.

Equipment required
None

Common competencies

CC1 History taking
CC2 Clinical examination
CC3 Therapeutics and safe prescribing
CC4 Time management and decision-making
CC5 Decision-making and clinical reasoning
CC6 Patient as the central focus of care
CC7 Prioritization of patient safety in clinical practice
CC12 Relationship with patients and communication

Paediatric major presentations (PMPs)

PMP6 Unconscious child

Paediatric acute presentations (PAPs)

PAP9 Fever in all age groups

Mark scheme

Introduces self	1
Confirms Adam's mother's identity	1
Explains diagnosis of febrile convulsion secondary to viral upper respiratory tract infection	2
Explains treatment consists of observation	2
Explains it is a very common condition	2
Advises convulsion caused by rapid increase in temperature	2
Advises no way to prevent future convulsions	2
Explains prognosis:	
• No direct link to epilepsy	1
• May recur	1
• No neurological sequelae	1
Invites questions	1
Provides safety net and written information about febrile convulsions	2
Shows non-verbal communication skills	2
Global score from examiner	5
Global score from actor	5
Total	**30**

Question 79 Poisoning

Instructions for candidate
Ambulance control has phoned to say they are bringing in a woman who has been found collapsed in her flat by friends. She has an empty bottle of antidepressants next to her. You have an experienced ED nurse with you. Please assess the patient and give any treatment required.

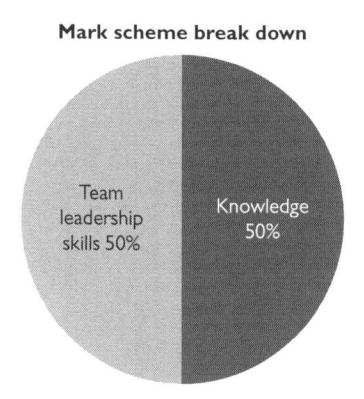

Mark scheme break down

- Team leadership skills 50%
- Knowledge 50%

Instructions for actor
You are an experienced ED nurse. You have basic airway skills; you can do bloods, get IV access, and do blood gases. Do not prompt the candidate.

Instructions for examiner
You may provide the candidate with the following information if requested:

A—secretions in mouth, improve with suctioning
B—RR 28, good air entry throughout, SaO_2 88%
C—HR 160 (ventricular tachycardia (VT)), BP 80/60, peripherally vasodilated, CRT 5 seconds
D—GCS 8 (E2, V2, M4), temperature 36.8°C, no focal neurology, pupils dilated but reactive

If the candidate requests that they want to intubate the patient, advise them that the equipment is being made ready and the anaesthetist will do this for them. After initial assessment, tell the candidate that the patient is having a tonic-clonic seizure. The seizure only stops if the candidate administers sodium bicarbonate. The following blood gas can be provided:

pH 7.1
pCO_2 12 kPa
pO_2 10 kPa
BE –18 mmol/L
Lactate 6 mmol/L

Equipment required
Standard adult resuscitation equipment (see introductory section)

Curriculum mapping
Sections of the CEM (2010) curriculum relevant to this question include the following.

Common competencies

CC1 History taking
CC2 Clinical examination
CC4 Time management and decision-making
CC5 Decision-making and clinical reasoning
CC6 Patient as the central focus of care
CC7 Prioritization of patient safety in clinical practice
CC8 Team work and patient safety
CC15 Communication with colleagues and cooperation

ACCS Major presentations CT1&2

CMP5 Shocked patient
CMP6 Unconscious atient

ACCS Acute presentations CT1&2

CAP27 Poisoning
CAP35 Ventilatory support

Guidelines available

http://www.collemergencymed.ac.uk/shop-floor/clinicalguidelines/, then follow **Tricyclic Antidepressant Overdose**

Mark scheme

Follows A B C D E approach	2
Calls for senior EM/anaesthetic/ITU assistance early	1
Assesses airway	1
Suctions airway (+/− uses airway adjuncts)	1
Assesses breathing	1
Gives high flow oxygen	1
Assesses circulation	1
Obtains IV access and bloods	1
Obtains VBG/ABG including blood glucose	1
Requests cardiac monitoring	1
Identifies rhythm on monitor as VT (with pulse)	1
Gives:	
• IV fluid bolus	1
• IV sodium bicarbonate 50ml of 8.4%	1
• Synchronized direct current (DC) shock	1
Applies 12-lead ECG	1
Reassesses patient	1
Does blood gas	1
Manages seizures:	
• Maintains airway	1

Continued

Question 79 Poisoning

Continued

• Gives IV sodium bicarbonate 50mL of 8.4%	1
• Requests RSI	1
Recognizes intensive care bed required	1
Displays team leadership skills	2
Global score from examiner	5
Total	**29**

Question 80 Mental state examination

Instructions for candidate
This patient has been brought to the ED after having been found wandering around in the street in a confused state. Please perform a mini mental state examination.

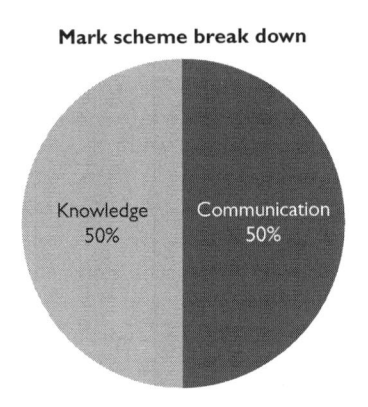

Mark scheme break down

- Knowledge 50%
- Communication 50%

Instructions for actor
You are very confused. You cannot answer any of the doctor's questions which test your orientation, e.g. 'Where are we now?' You cannot copy or draw anything that the doctor asks. But you can answer the other questions.

Instructions for examiner
Observation only.

Equipment required
Paper, pen, pencil

Curriculum mapping
Sections of the CEM (2010) curriculum relevant to this question include the following.

Common competencies

CC1 History taking
CC5 Decision-making and clinical reasoning
CC6 Patient as the central focus of care
CC7 Prioritization of patient safety in clinical practice
CC11 Management of long-term conditions and promoting patient self-care
CC12 Relationship with patients and communication

ACCS Acute presentations CT1&2

CAP30 Mental health

Question 80 Mental state examination

Mark scheme

Introduces self	2
Checks identity	1
Explains needs to ask a series of questions	1
Tests orientation with the following questions:	½ mark for each (max 5)
1. What is today's date?	
2. What is the month?	
3. What is the year?	
4. What day of the week is it today?	
5. What season is it?	
6. What is the name of this clinic (place)?	
7. What floor are we on?	
8. What city are we in?	
9. What county are we in?	
10. What country are we in?	
Tests immediate recall, e.g. ball, flag, tree	1
Tests attention, e.g. spell WORLD backwards or subtract serial sevens from 100 (one only)	1
Tests delayed verbal recall with three objects given previously	1
Tests naming two objects, e.g. watch, pencil	1
Tests repetition by asking patient to repeat 'no ifs, ands, or buts'	1
Tests three-stage command, e.g. 'take this piece of paper, fold it in half, and put it on the table'	1
Tests reading with command 'close your eyes'	1
Tests writing by asking patient to write a sentence	1
Tests copying by asking patient to copy two pentagons	1
Is patient and reassuring throughout	2
Correctly scores patient's answers and grades severity	2
Global score from examiner	5
Global score from actor	5
Total	**32**

Question 81 Sepsis

Instructions for candidate
You are called to resus to see a 62-year-old woman who has been unwell all day today with fevers and shivers. She had an endoscopic retrograde cholangiopancreatography (ERCP) as a day case yesterday. You have an experienced nurse from the ED with you. Please assess the patient and treat as necessary.

Mark scheme break down

- Team leadership skills 50%
- Knowledge 50%

Instructions for actor 1 (patient)
You had an ERCP yesterday because you have been having problems with gallstones. You felt fine when you went home from hospital but overnight you felt hot and sweaty. All day today you have been getting worse, with fevers and vomiting, and now you feel really awful. You have a bad headache and pain in the upper abdomen. You are normally fit and well. Apart from gallstones you have no medical problems, and take no medication and have no allergies. You work as a secretary and live with your husband, who is at work.

Instructions for actor 2 (nurse)
You are a staff nurse in the ED. You know where all the equipment is kept and can hand it to the candidate, but you don't act without being clearly instructed to do so.

Instructions for examiner
You may provide the candidate with the following information if requested:

A—patent, patient-speaking
B—reasonable air entry, SaO_2 90% on air, poor trace, 92% on 15 L oxygen, RR 28
C—HR 130, BP 90/70, peripherally vasodilated, CRT 3 seconds
D—GCS 14, very anxious

Temperature 39°C
Erythematous skin all over

There is no improvement in BP despite 3 L of fluid. If the candidate gives more fluid than this, the patient becomes very confused and drowsy (to simulate cerebral oedema). If the candidate mentions intubation, tell the candidate that the kit can be set up, but that the anaesthetist will intubate when they arrive.

Equipment required
Standard adult resuscitation equipment (see introductory section)

Question 81 Sepsis

Curriculum mapping

Sections of the CEM (2010) curriculum relevant to this question include the following.

Common competencies

CC1 History taking
CC2 Clinical examination
CC3 Therapeutics and safe prescribing
CC4 Time management and decision-making
CC5 Decision-making and clinical reasoning
CC8 Team work and patient safety
CC10 Infection control
CC15 Communication with colleagues and cooperation

ACCS Major presentations CT1&2

CMP4 Septic patient
CMP5 Shocked patient

Mark scheme

Introduces self to patient	1
Follows A B C D E approach	2
Calls for senior EM/anaesthetic/ITU assistance early	1
Assesses airway	1
Assesses breathing	1
Gives high flow oxygen	1
Assesses circulation	1
Recognizes and mentions severe sepsis as probable diagnosis	1
Ensures IV access with bloods and blood gas	3
Specifically mentions blood cultures	1
Gives IV fluid bolus promptly	1
Reassesses and repeats fluid bolus	2
Checks temperature	1
Examines for source of sepsis	1
Requests CXR to identify source of sepsis	1
Requests urine sample for MCS to identify source of sepsis	1
Requests urinary catheterization	1
Gives broad-spectrum IV antibiotics	1
Recognizes need for ITU/pressors/inotropes/intubation when no improvement	2
Mentions sepsis care bundles/'sepsis six'/'surviving sepsis' including:	
• Central line with mixed venous SaO_2	1
• Goal-directed therapy	1
Displays team leadership skills	2
Global score from examiner	5
Global score from actors	5
Total	**38**

Question 82 ECG

Instructions for candidate
You have a third-year medical student who has asked you to explain how to read an ECG.

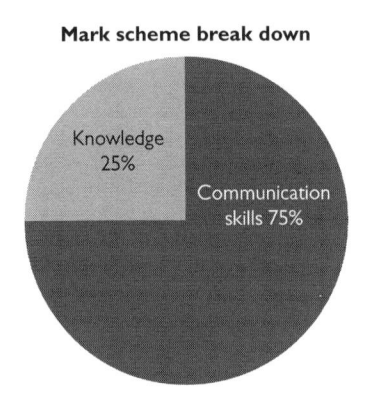

Mark scheme break down

- Knowledge 25%
- Communication skills 75%

Instructions for actor
You are a third-year medical student who is attached to the ED for the week. You have never been taught how to read an ECG before, but you have heard doctors talking about them. You are able to follow the candidate's instructions. Do not do anything that they have not instructed you to do.

Instructions for examiner
Observation only.

Equipment required
ECGs (normal)

Curriculum mapping
Sections of the CEM (2010) curriculum relevant to this question include the following.

Common competencies

CC15 Communication with colleagues and cooperation
CC23 Teaching and training

Mark scheme

Establishes what student already knows	1
Explains indications for ECGs	2
Follows structured approach to ECG interpretation	2
Explains anatomical considerations:	
• Territories including inferior, anterior, and lateral	1
• How lead positions correlate to anatomy	1

Continued

Question 82 ECG

Continued

Explains how to identify electrical activity	1
Explains P waves	1
Explains QRS waves	1
Explains QRS length	1
Explains T waves	1
Explains PR interval	1
Explains QT interval	1
Explains axis	1
Explains relevance of squared paper	2
Explains how to calculate rate	1
Describes simple conduction problems	1
Describes simple ST problems	1
Describes simple arrhythmias	1
Closure—reviews learning with student	1
Invites questions	1
Suggests follow–up, e.g. look at ECG on every patient, meet again to recap	1
Demonstrates systematic, organized approach	2
Global score from examiner	5
Global score from actor	5
Total	**36**

Question 83 Deep vein thrombosis

Instructions for candidate
You have a new Foundation Year 2 doctor (F2) in the ED today who has just seen a woman with a swollen leg. They have asked you how to investigate suspected deep vein thrombosis (DVT). Please explain how to assess a patient's risk for having a DVT.

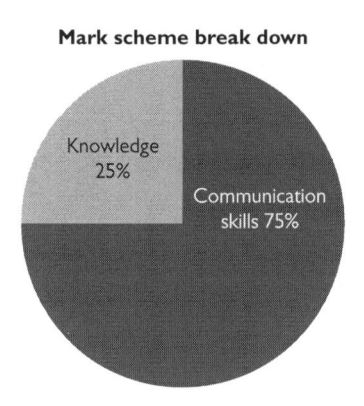

Mark scheme break down

- Knowledge 25%
- Communication skills 75%

Instructions for actor
You are a new F2 in ED for the week. You have never seen a patient with a swollen leg before. Your patient is a young fit woman who hurt her leg playing squash yesterday and has some pain and swelling in the back of her calf today. The triage nurse has given her some paracetamol and the pain is a bit better. She has no medical problems, is not on any medication, and has never had a DVT before. You are able to follow the candidate's instructions. Do not do anything that they have not instructed you to do.

Instructions for examiner
Observation only.

Equipment required
None

Curriculum mapping
Sections of the CEM (2010) curriculum relevant to this question include the following.

Common competencies

CC15 Communication with colleagues and cooperation
CC23 Teaching and training

Mark scheme

Introduces self	1
Explores what F2 already knows	1
Explains concept of screening test (rule in, rule out)	2
Explains risk factors (Well's criteria):	
• Active cancer?	1
• Bedridden recently > 3 days or major surgery within 4 weeks?	1

Continued

Question 83 Deep vein thrombosis

Continued

• Calf swelling > 3 cm compared to other leg?	1
• Collateral (non-varicose) superficial veins present?	1
• Entire leg swollen?	1
• Localized tenderness along deep venous system?	1
• Pitting oedema, greater in symptomatic leg?	1
• Paralysis, paresis, or recent plaster immobilization of lower extremity?	1
• Previously documented DVT?	1
Explains if another diagnosis is more likely, then 2 is taken off total score	1
Explains scoring system—one for each point above	1
Explains high, medium, and low risk outcomes	1
Explains management of each group	2
Explains alternative diagnoses including Achilles' tendon tear, muscular pain	2
Discusses individual patient and makes a management plan	2
Suggests ways of gaining more skills	1
Closure—reviews learning with F2	1
Demonstrates systematic, organized approach	2
Global score from examiner	5
Global score from actor	5
Total	**36**

Question 84 Breaking bad news 4

Instructions for candidate
You are taking over the care of a patient (a 55-year-old male) from a colleague who has gone off shift. He had arranged a CT scan of the patient's head as they had fallen over in the street, hit their head, and had a seizure. The patient has just returned from scan and the CT scan showed some ring-enhancing lesions within the brain compatible with cerebral metastases. Please discuss the results with him.

Mark scheme break down

- Knowledge 25%
- Communication skills 75%

Instructions for actor
You are a normally fit and well 55 year old, who has smoked heavily for 40 years. You have had headaches off and on over the past few weeks, but have been under stress at work. On the way to the bus stop after work you collapsed to the ground and have no recollection of events until you arrived in hospital. You want to know the alternative diagnoses and what can be done about it.

Instructions for examiner
Observation only.

Equipment required
Relevant CT scan

Curriculum mapping
Sections of the CEM (2010) curriculum relevant to this question include the following.

Common competencies

CC6 Patient as the central focus of care
CC12 Relationship with patients and communication
CC13 Breaking bad news
CC15 Communication with colleagues and cooperation

ACCS Acute presentations CT1&2

CAP18 Head injury

Question 84 Breaking bad news 4

Mark scheme

Introduces self to patient and explains role	2
Asks if can have nurse present, bleep/phone switched off, department matron/sister aware of location	2
Checks what has happened and what patient knows so far	2
Explains what CT scan shows and demonstrates CT	3
Explains need for further investigation such as looking for primary cancer	2
Gives patient opportunity to ask questions and answers appropriately	2
Summarizes	1
Offers to call relatives/friends	1
Global score from examiner	5
Global score from actor	5
Total	**25**

Question 85 Aortic aneurysm

Instructions for candidate

This patient, John Smith, is known to have a 7-cm infra-renal aortic aneurysm. He is awaiting an elective endovascular repair at the local vascular centre. He has presented today after collapsing in the garden with abdominal pain. A FAST scan done by your colleague confirms the aneurysm and shows free fluid in the abdomen. His observations are as follows:

HR 128
BP 80/54
RR 32

The ambulance crew have managed to get wide-bore IV access in both arms. His medical details and observation chart are provided for you. His pain has been controlled with 2.5 mg of IV morphine, and IV fluids have been withheld.

Please arrange his transfer to the vascular centre nearby (5 miles away) by telephone. Your hospital does not have a vascular service. If you pick up the telephone, you will be able to talk to the vascular registrar on call.

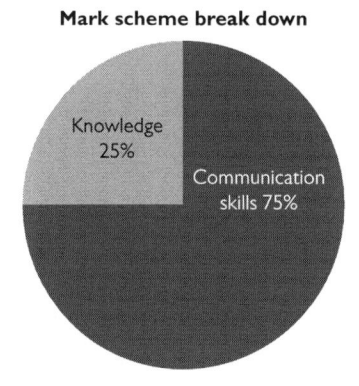

Mark scheme break down

- Knowledge 25%
- Communication skills 75%

Instructions for actor

You are the vascular surgery registrar on call, Mr Jones. You are in the regional vascular centre at St John's Hospital. The candidate will refer a very unwell patient to you. They will not have details such as CT results or blood gases. You can ask for these results (they should not have done these tests because it may delay the transfer). You want to know all the patient's medical details and make sure that it is appropriate to transfer this patient.

You should ask if they have got IV access and what IV fluids they have had (the candidate should say that they have not been given fluids because the BP is adequate ('permissive hypotension')). You accept the transfer. Ask the patient to be sent to the emergency theatre suite at St John's Hospital.

Instructions for examiner

Observation only.

Equipment

Telephone
Medical charts with the following information:

- Drug chart with IV morphine prescribed
- Patient details:
  - Mr John Smith
  - Date of birth 02/02/1933
  - Hospital number T1120332
- Medical history:
  - Hypertension
  - Ex-smoker
  - Type 2 diabetes (diet controlled)
- Medication:
  - Bendroflumethiazide
  - No allergies
- Social history:
  - Widowed. Independent
  - Family live nearby
- Observations:
  - Alert, GCS 15
  - HR 128
  - BP 80/54
  - RR 32
  - ECG—sinus tachycardia
  - Temperature 37.2°C

Curriculum mapping

Sections of the CEM (2010) curriculum relevant to this question include the following.

Common competencies

CC4 Time management and decision-making
CC5 Decision-making and clinical reasoning
CC6 Patient as the central focus of care
CC7 Prioritization of patient safety in clinical practice
CC8 Team work and patient safety
CC15 Communication with colleagues and cooperation
CC18 Valid consent

ACCS Major presentations CT1&2

CMP4 Septic patient
CMP5 Shocked patient
CMP6 Unconscious patient

ACCS Acute presentations CT1&2

CAP1 Abdominal pain including loin pain
CAP32 Syncope and presyncope

Guidelines available

http://www.collemergencymed.ac.uk/shop-floor/clinicalguidelines/, then follow **Transfer and Management of Patients with a Diagnosis of Ruptured Abdominal Aortic Aneurysm**

Self-Assessment for the MCEM Part C

Mark scheme

Introduces self	1
Checks speaking with vascular registrar and takes name	1
States clearly that patient needs to be transferred	1
Provides brief history	2
Includes ultrasound findings	2
Describes observations in brief history	2
Corrects details in history when prompted	2
Makes it clear that patient is very unwell	1
Asks where to transfer patient within hospital	1
Confirms bed available	1
Asks if anything else required	2
Declines getting a CT scan (to avoid delay)	1
Declines giving IV fluids (permissive hypotension)	1
Confirms will arrange ambulance urgently	1
Global score from examiner	5
Global score from actor	5
Total	**29**

Question 86 Central line

Instructions for candidate

This 21-year-old IV drug user, Chloe, has presented to the ED with a 24-hour history of severe abdominal pain and vomiting. Chloe tells you she is an alcoholic and has had pancreatitis in the past, and now has diabetes because her pancreas has been destroyed. She looks pale and sweaty, with a BP of 80/60 and HR of 120.

She has no accessible peripheral veins, even with the aid of ultrasound, and needs IV fluids. Please insert an internal jugular central venous access line into the model provided. The actor will play the role of Chloe, but the central line should be inserted into the model.

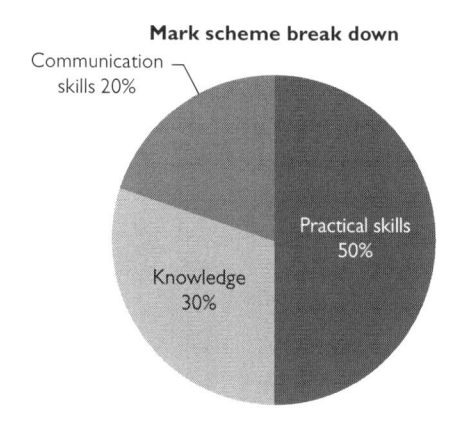

Mark scheme break down
- Communication skills 20%
- Knowledge 30%
- Practical skills 50%

Instructions for actor

You have been brought to hospital by ambulance with severe abdominal pain and vomiting. You have had pancreatitis in the past and it feels like the same thing. Your veins have disappeared from injecting drugs for several years. At present, you inject into your neck veins. On the last few times you were in hospital, you have had to have central lines. You know what is involved and go along with what the candidate advises.

Instructions for examiner

Ensure that the candidate is aware they should carry out the procedure on the model, not the actor. When the candidate indicates that they would like to wash their hands and use personal protective equipment, tell them to proceed without actually doing so, to save time. Do not award a mark for this if the candidate does not mention it.

Equipment required

Model for central line access
Cleaning solution
Sterile gloves, gown, and mask
Gauze swabs
Ultrasound machine
Local anaesthetic
Sterile saline
Selection of needles and syringes

Self-Assessment for the MCEM Part C

Introducers
Guide wire
Scalpel
Central venous catheter
Sutures

Curriculum mapping

Sections of the CEM (2010) curriculum relevant to this question include the following.

Common competencies

CC4 Time management and decision-making
CC7 Prioritization of patient safety in clinical practice
CC10 Infection control

ACCS Major presentations CT1&2

CMP4 Septic patient
CMP5 Shocked patient

ACCS Acute presentations CT1&2

CAP1 Abdominal pain including loin pain

Mark scheme

Introduces self	1
Checks identity	1
Explains procedure	2
Obtains verbal consent, assent	1
Gathers correct equipment	2
Ensures correct patient position	1
Uses sterile technique (washes hands, uses gown, gloves, and mask)	1
Flushes line with saline	1
Uses ultrasound to identify anatomy or in real time	1
Gives local anaesthetic	1
Identifies internal jugular vein with needle and syringe by aspirating blood	1
Introduces guide wire	1
Opens track with introducers and scalpel to skin	1
Positions catheter, maintaining hold on wire throughout	1
Aspirates and flushes catheter ports	1
Secures catheter with sutures	1
Applies dressing	1
Allows patient to sit up, reassures, offers painkillers	1
Thanks patient	1
Clears sharps	2
Global score from examiner	5
Global score from actor	5
Total	**33**

Question 87 Asystole

Instructions for candidate
You are called to resus to see a 75-year-old woman who has been found collapsed in her nursing home. You have an experienced nurse from the ED with you. Please assess the patient and treat as necessary.

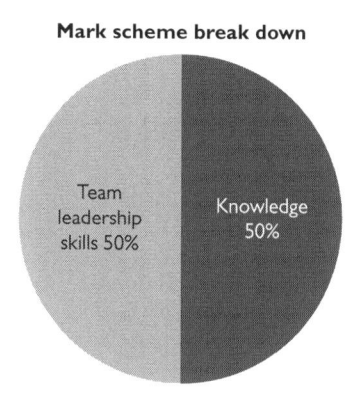

Mark scheme break down

- Team leadership skills 50%
- Knowledge 50%

Instructions for actor
You are a staff nurse in the ED. You know where all the equipment is kept and can hand it to the candidate, but you don't act without being clearly instructed to do so.

Instructions for examiner
You may provide the candidate with the following information if requested:

A—clear airway, tolerates airway adjuncts
B—apnoeic, unable to measure SaO_2
C—no palpable pulse or signs of life, asystole on monitor
D—GCS 3
No response to resuscitation

The candidate is expected to terminate resuscitation after 5 rounds of time-accelerated CPR cycles.

Equipment required
Standard adult resuscitation equipment (see introductory section)

Curriculum mapping
Sections of the CEM (2010) curriculum relevant to this question include the following.

Common competencies
CC1 History taking
CC2 Clinical examination
CC3 Therapeutics and safe prescribing
CC4 Time management and decision-making
CC5 Decision-making and clinical reasoning
CC6 Patient as the central focus of care

CC7 Prioritization of patient safety in clinical practice
CC8 Team work and patient safety
CC12 Relationship with patients and communication
CC13 Breaking bad news
CC15 Communication with colleagues and cooperation

ACCS Major presentations CT1&2

CMP2 Cardiorespiratory arrest
CMP5 Shocked patient

ACCS Acute presentations CT1&2

CAP6 Breathlessness
CAP35 Ventilatory support

Guidelines available

http://www.resus.org.uk/pages/alsalgo.pdf

Mark scheme

Gives oxygen	1
Follows sequential A B C D E approach	2
Calls for anaesthetic/senior assistance	1
Promptly diagnoses cardiac arrest	1
Recognizes asystole	1
Promptly starts CPR	1
Carries out early intubation	1
Carries out early IV access	1
Gives adequate CPR	1
Gives adrenaline	1
Considers '4 Hs' and '4 Ts'	4
Considers giving fluids	1
Realizes futility of situation	1
Discusses stopping resuscitation with the team	1
Stops resuscitation	1
Asks to talk to patient's next of kin	1
Considers team debrief	1
Displays team leadership skills	2
Global score from examiner	5
Total	**28**

Question 88 Facial wound

Instructions for candidate

This 8-year-old has fallen over in the playground at school and cut her face. She has a 1-cm wound to the lateral aspect of her left eyebrow. She is otherwise fine. Using the model, please close the wound using tissue adhesive.

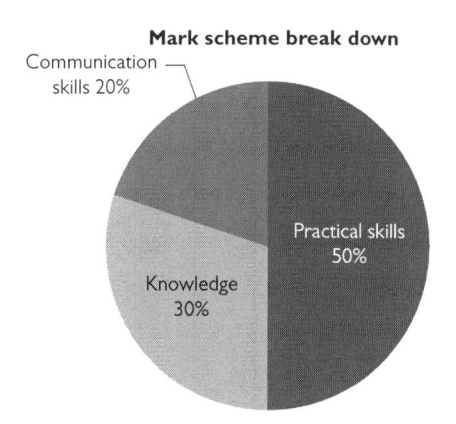

Mark scheme break down

- Communication skills 20%
- Practical skills 50%
- Knowledge 30%

Instructions for examiner

Observation only.

Equipment required

Model representing facial laceration
Cleaning solution
Sterile gloves
Gauze swabs
Local anaesthetic
Sterile saline
Selection of needles and syringes
Tissue glue
Dressings

Curriculum mapping

Sections of the CEM (2010) curriculum relevant to this question include the following.

Common competencies

CC2 Clinical examination
CC3 Therapeutics and safe prescribing
CC5 Decision-making and clinical reasoning
CC6 Patient as the central focus of care
CC10 Infection control
CC12 Relationship with patients and communication

Paediatric acute presentations (PAPs)

PAP15 Pain in children

Self-Assessment for the MCEM Part C

Mark scheme

Introduces self	1
Washes hands	1
Checks analgesia given	1
Ensures parent/guardian present	1
Ensures paediatric trained nurse/play specialist present	1
Asks parents/guardians about tetanus	1
Explains procedure	2
Asks about previous scar formation, e.g. keloid problems	1
Invites questions about procedure/technique	1
Selects tissue glue	1
Uses clean technique	1
Ensures thorough saline lavage	1
Uses correct glue technique:	
• Closely opposes wound edges	1
• Applies glue to skin surface	1
Warns to keep dry	1
Discusses that glue will normally separate from skin at 8–10 days	1
Warns about signs of infection	1
Advises when to return if worried and provides written information sheet/leaflet	1
Advises there will still be a scar	1
Invites questions	1
Global score from examiner	5
Global score from actor	5
Total	**31**

Question 89 Dehydration

Instructions for candidate

This 2-year-old child, Joe, has had diarrhoea and vomiting for the last 48 hours. Joe has been brought to the ED by his parents because they are concerned about dehydration. You have assessed Joe, and he has mild signs of dehydration but is still vomiting. You would like to start an oral fluid regime on the child. Please explain this to the parents.

Mark scheme break down

- Knowledge 25%
- Communication skills 75%

Instructions for actor

You are the mother of a toddler, Joe, who has had diarrhoea and vomiting for the last 2 days. You have tried giving him water, milk, juice, and fizzy drinks at home, but he keeps being sick. He has had five episodes of watery stool since the illness began. He has been alert throughout, but is miserable and off his food. He has not had any floppy episodes. He is normally fit and well, with no medical problems.

Before coming to hospital, you spoke to a friend who had a child in a similar situation recently, who came to hospital and the child was given fluids through a drip. You want to know why your child cannot have the same treatment. After receiving a thorough explanation about the oral fluid regime, you agree that your child can try it.

Instructions for examiner

Observation only.

Equipment required

None

Curriculum mapping

Sections of the CEM (2010) curriculum relevant to this question include the following.

Common competencies

CC1 History taking
CC4 Time management and decision-making
CC6 Patient as the central focus of care
CC12 Relationship with patients and communication

Paediatric acute presentations (PAPs)

PAP1 Abdominal pain
PAP7 Dehydration secondary to diarrhoea and vomiting
PAP9 Fever in all age groups

Self-Assessment for the MCEM Part C

Mark scheme

Introduces self	1
Confirms Joe's mother's identity	2
Explains diagnosis of gastroenteritis	2
Explains treatment consists of oral fluid regime and what this involves, and what the reasoning behind this approach is, including NICE guidance	3
Answers mother's questions about oral fluids	2
Explains why IV fluids not recommended	2
Deals adequately with concerns	3
Remains professional and polite when challenged	2
Invites questions	1
Provides safety net +/− patient information sheet/leaflet	1
Shows non-verbal communication skills	2
Global score from examiner	5
Global score from actor	5
Total	**31**

Question 90 Needlestick injury

Instructions for candidate
You are the ED registrar on nights when your Senior House Officer (SHO) tells you they have received a needlestick injury from a patient whilst cannulating. They are very concerned and have come to you for advice.

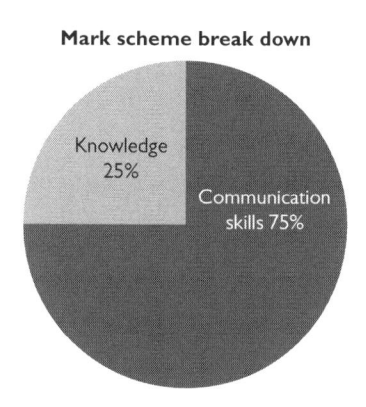

Mark scheme break down

- Knowledge 25%
- Communication skills 75%

Instructions for actor
You are a junior doctor in the ED. You have been looking after an elderly lady who has a fractured neck of femur (NOF) after falling at home. While putting a cannula in, the patient moved her arm suddenly and you sustained a needlestick injury from the cannula into the tip of your right index finger.

You have washed it under the tap and have now come to ask your registrar for advice. You are very worried about contracting HIV. You have had all the recommended immunizations and blood tests, through your hospital occupational health department, and you are completely up to date. The patient is an elderly lady with hypertension and diabetes and no other medical problems.

Instructions for examiner
Observation only.

Equipment required
None

Curriculum mapping
Sections of the CEM (2010) curriculum relevant to this question include the following.

Common competencies
CC1 History taking
CC3 Therapeutics and safe prescribing
CC4 Time management and decision-making
CC5 Decision-making and clinical reasoning
CC6 Patient as the central focus of care
CC7 Prioritization of patient safety in clinical practice

CC8 Team work and patient safety
CC9 Principles of safety and quality improvement
CC10 Infection control
CC14 Complaints and medical error
CC15 Communication with colleagues and cooperation
CC16 Health promotion and public health
CC17 Ethics and confidentiality

Mark scheme

Introduces self	1
Establishes story	2
Establishes good rapport	1
Establishes first aid measures undertaken	1
Explains very low risk of blood-borne virus transmission	1
Explains need to establish risk from patient (mentions at least 2 of blood transfusions, known HIV/Hep, IV drug users, sexual partners of high-risk groups)	2
Explains need to establish risk from type of injury (e.g. hollow needle containing blood)	2
Checks immunization status	1
Explains needs blood tests from recipient	2
Explains needs blood tests from donor:	
• With consent	1
• Not to be done by junior doctor	1
Explains needs occupational health follow-up	1
Checks cannulation technique	1
Explains reasons for wearing gloves for cannulation	1
Ensures incident reporting has happened	1
Invites questions	1
Checks to see if junior doctor feels comfortable to continue shift	1
Summarizes	1
Global score from examiner	5
Global score from actor	5
Total	**32**

Question 91 Blood gas analysis

Instructions for candidate
Please teach this final-year medical student how to interpret these arterial blood gas results:

pH 7.01
pO_2 21 kPa
pCO_2 12 kPa
HCO_3 23 mEq/L
Base excess −1 mmol/L

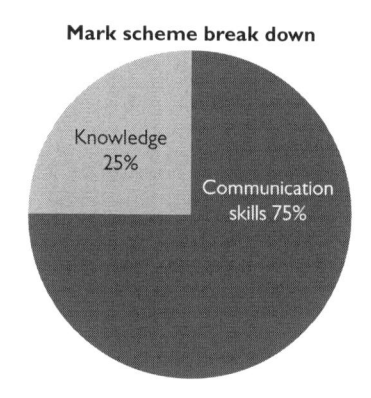

Mark scheme break down

- Knowledge 25%
- Communication skills 75%

Instructions for actor
You are a final-year medical student in the ED. You have been working with the team in resus looking after a patient who has had a return of spontaneous circulation after an out-of-hospital cardiac arrest. He has had an arterial blood gas taken. You ask the registrar to explain what the results mean. You have learned about blood gas measurements in theory but have not had the chance to analyse one from a real patient before.

Instructions for examiner
Observation only.

Equipment required
Abnormal arterial blood gas result

Curriculum mapping
Sections of the CEM (2010) curriculum relevant to this question include the following.

Common competencies
CC5 Decision-making and clinical reasoning
CC23 Teaching and training

Mark scheme

Introduces self	1
Establishes student's previous knowledge/understanding of the topic	1
Establishes good rapport	1
Introduces topic and explains its importance in the clinical setting	1
Sets objectives	1
Demonstrates systematic approach, explaining normal values and implication of high or low result of the following:	
• pH	1
• Respiratory component	1
• Metabolic component	1
• Compensation	1
Diagnoses example result	2
Relates result to clinical picture	1
Questions student to assess understanding	1
Invites student to ask questions	2
Summarizes learning points	1
Encourages/directs further study/learning opportunities	1
Demonstrates systematic, organized approach	2
Global score from examiner	5
Global score from actor	5
Total	**29**

Question 92 Jaundice

Instructions for candidate
Please take a history from this 30-year-old man presenting with jaundice.

Mark scheme break down
- Communication skills 20%
- Knowledge 80%

Instructions for actor
You are a 30-year-old man. You have felt unwell for about 2 months. Initially you had aching joints and muscles, which you thought was flu. But in the last 2 days you have developed yellow skin and eyes, and you feel very unwell. Your stool and urine have been normal in colour. You have lost a stone in weight, slowly over the last year.

You are a heavy drinker. You drink about 6 pints every day, often followed by several glasses of vodka. You used to inject heroin, but you are currently on a methadone programme. You have never had tests for HIV or hepatitis. You don't have any other medical problems or take any other drugs. You smoke 20 cigarettes a day. You are unemployed but you used to work as a builder. You were recently sacked when you came into work drunk. You are divorced and live alone. You have never travelled outside the UK, never had a blood transfusion, and never had sexual contacts with prostitutes or homosexuals.

Instructions for examiner
Observation only.

Equipment required
None

Curriculum mapping
Sections of the CEM (2010) curriculum relevant to this question include the following.

Common competencies

CC1 History taking
CC4 Time management and decision-making
CC6 Patient as the central focus of care
CC12 Relationship with patients and communication

ACCS Acute presentations CT1&2

CAP19 Jaundice

Self-Assessment for the MCEM Part C

Mark scheme

Introduces self	1
Establishes reason for attendance	2
Takes thorough history of presenting complaint—duration, nature, previous jaundice, associated symptoms	4
Asks about risk factors for infective hepatitis:	
• Travel	1
• Sexual contacts	1
• IV drug use	1
• Blood transfusions	1
Asks about alcohol history	2
Asks about stool and urine changes	2
Obtains medication history	2
Asks about allergy history	1
Asks about immunization history	1
Obtains past medical history	1
Asks about social history	1
Invites questions	1
Summarizes history	1
Suggests next steps/action in management of the patient	1
Global score from examiner	5
Global score from actor	5
Total	**35**

Question 93 Driving advice

Instructions for candidate

You have just seen a patient who has attended the ED several times with seizures, thought to be due to alcohol withdrawal. He has now recovered and is ready to be discharged. Today he tells you that he has just got a new job as a delivery driver. Please discuss the issue of driving with the patient before he leaves the department.

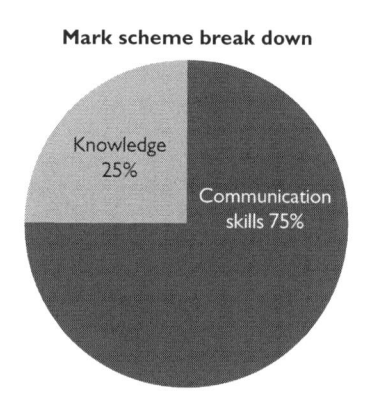

Mark scheme break down

- Knowledge 25%
- Communication skills 75%

Instructions for actor

You are a 50-year-old man. You are a heavy drinker. You drink about 8 pints of cider every day. You started drinking after the breakdown of your marriage 10 years ago. You have tried to stop drinking several times, but each time you do, you have a seizure. You have been told by doctors that it is important not to suddenly stop alcohol. You have recently seen your GP to get some help, and you are on the waiting list for a referral to the Drug and Alcohol Support Team in your area.

You don't have any other medical problems or take any other drugs. You smoke 20 cigarettes a day. You have been unemployed for years but have recently started driving a delivery van to help a friend out 3 days a week. This is an unofficial job, for which you are paid in cash—which you badly need. You are divorced and live alone. You do sometimes drink in the morning but you 'don't drink much' on the days that you go to work. You have never had a fit when you've been behind the wheel. You refuse to consider that driving is dangerous in your condition. You refuse to tell the DVLA or discuss it with your GP and want to leave the department.

Instructions for examiner

Observation only.

Equipment required

None

Curriculum mapping

Sections of the CEM (2010) curriculum relevant to this question include the following.

Common competencies

CC1 History taking
CC5 Decision-making and clinical reasoning
CC6 Patient as the central focus of care

CC7 Prioritization of patient safety in clinical practice
CC12 Relationship with patients and communication
CC13 Breaking bad news
CC16 Health promotion and public health
CC17 Ethics and confidentiality

ACCS Acute presentations CT1&2

CAP15 Fits/seizure

Guidelines available

http://www.collemergencymed.ac.uk/shop-floor/clinicalguidelines/, then follow **CEM Summary of DVLA Fitness to Drive Medical Standards**

Mark scheme

Introduces self	1
Establishes diagnosis—alcohol withdrawal seizures, ready for discharge, follow-up with GP	2
Advises about not suddenly stopping alcohol	4
Introduces topic of work as a driver	4
Explains risk of driving with seizures and alcohol use	2
Advises they should stop driving immediately	2
Appeals to patient to stop and inform DVLA	2
Advises patient that driving after a seizure invalidates car insurance and life insurance	1
Advises patient that they could be criminally liable should they be involved in a road accident	1
Informs patient that doctors must inform DVLA even without patient's consent in such a case	1
Offers to write to GP and to Drug/Alcohol Support Team to attempt to expedite appointment	1
Global score from examiner	5
Global score from actor	5
Total	**31**

Question 94 Haematemesis

Instructions for candidate

Please take a history from this patient who has presented with a history of vomiting blood. He is haemodynamically stable and comfortable at present. He has been seen by the triage nurse who has sent off blood tests and has inserted a wide-bore cannula. His observations are as follows:

HR 68
BP 130/88
RR 14
Temperature 37.6°C

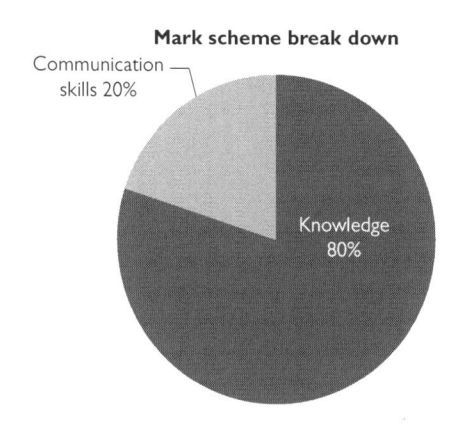

Mark scheme break down

- Communication skills 20%
- Knowledge 80%

Instructions for actor

You are a 40-year-old man who smokes 10 cigarettes a day. You have been under a lot of pressure at work lately (you are a lawyer). You have been getting indigestion-type pains most days for the last month. They are a burning, severe pain in the middle of your upper abdomen. They improve when you take antacid medication.

You drink a 'few glasses of wine' (more like a bottle) most evenings whilst working in your study, and find this is the only way you can switch off. Today the pain got particularly bad, and you vomited up a small amount of fresh red blood. You have not noticed any change to your stool or had any bleeding. You have never had any bleeding like this before. You are normally fit and well and don't take any regular medications. You take Nurofen™ for headaches 'most days'—you think these are stress-related headaches. You live with your wife and two children. You don't use any other drugs.

Instructions for examiner

Observation only.

Equipment required

None

Curriculum mapping

Sections of the CEM (2010) curriculum relevant to this question include the following.

Common competencies

CC1 History taking
CC12 Relationship with patients and communication

ACCS Acute presentations CT1&2

CAP16 Haematemesis and melaena

Mark scheme

Introduces self	1
Establishes reason for attendance	2
Takes thorough history of presenting complaint—duration, nature, amount of blood, associated symptoms	4
Asks about risk factors for bleeding:	
• Alcohol intake	1
• Medication—warfarin and other anticoagulants, steroid, NSAIDs	1
• Smoking	1
• Previous variceal bleeds	1
• Previous peptic ulcer disease	1
Takes medication history including specifically:	
• Anticoagulation	1
• Antiplatelet agents	1
Asks about past medical history	1
Asks about social history	1
Calculates Rockall score equals zero:	
• Age less than 60 years	1
• No evidence of shock (BP > 100 and HR < 100)	1
• No comorbidities	1
Summarizes history	1
Advises ongoing management includes physical examination, and upper GI endoscopy as an outpatient	1
Advises to see GP to discuss getting help with stress management	1
Advises stopping NSAIDs	1
Global score from examiner	5
Global score from actor	5
Total	**35**

Question 95 Intraosseus access

Instructions for candidate

You are involved in a paediatric resuscitation case. Please demonstrate the technique of IO access in a timely fashion, using the equipment available.

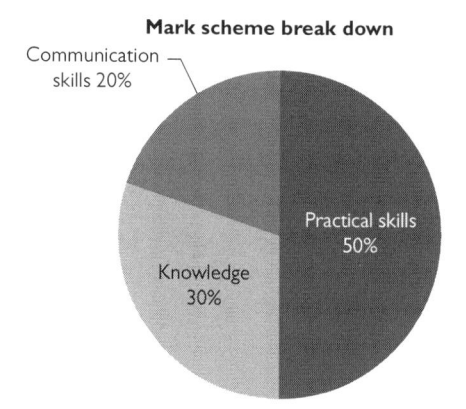

Mark scheme break down
- Communication skills 20%
- Knowledge 30%
- Practical skills 50%

Instructions for examiner

Ensure that the candidate is aware they should carry out the procedure on the model, not the actor. When the candidate indicates that they would like to wash their hands and use personal protective equipment, tell them to proceed without actually doing so, to save time. Do not award a mark for this if the candidate does not mention it.

Equipment required

Standard paediatric resuscitation equipment (see introductory section)
Paediatric manikin appropriate for use of IO needles

Curriculum mapping

Sections of the CEM (2010) curriculum relevant to this question include the following.

Common competencies

CC3 Therapeutics and safe prescribing
CC12 Relationship with patients and communication

Paediatric major presentations (PMPs)

PMP5 Shocked child
PMP6 Unconscious child

Mark scheme

Introduces self	1
Checks identity	1
Checks procedure explained to parents	1
Obtains verbal consent, assent	1

Continued

Continued

Gathers correct equipment (chooses equipment familiar to them from kit provided)	2
Ensures correct patient position	1
Follows aseptic technique	1
Flushes line with saline prior to use	1
Considers local anaesthetic	1
Ensures correct landmark—medial aspect of proximal tibia	1
Successfully sites needle and safely deals with trochar	1
Aspirates marrow and sends for glucose, cross match, and culture	1
Attaches connector	1
Flushes line	1
Secures to skin	1
Clears sharps	2
Demonstrates systematic, organized approach	2
Global score from examiner	5
Total	**25**

Question 96 Wound closure

Instructions for candidate
This 82-year-old has tripped over a rug in her living room. She has banged her shin and has sustained a large pretibial skin tear. She is otherwise fine. Using the model and the equipment available, please close the wound and explain any ongoing treatment needed.

Mark scheme break down
- Communication skills 20%
- Knowledge 30%
- Practical skills 50%

Instructions for examiner
Observation only.

Equipment required
Model representing pretibial laceration
Cleaning solution
Sterile gloves
Gauze swabs
Local anaesthetic
Sterile saline
Selection of needles and syringes
Tissue glue
Steristrips in selection of sizes
Dressings

Curriculum mapping
Sections of the CEM (2010) curriculum relevant to this question include the following.

Common competencies
CC1 History taking
CC2 Clinical examination
CC3 Therapeutics and safe prescribing
CC6 Patient as the central focus of care
CC7 Prioritization of patient safety in clinical practice
CC10 Infection control
CC11 Management of long-term conditions and promoting patient self-care
CC12 Relationship with patients and communication

Self-Assessment for the MCEM Part C

ACCS Acute presentations CT1&2

CAP23 Pain management
CAP33 Traumatic limb and joint injuries

Mark scheme

Introduces self	1
Washes hands	1
Checks analgesia given	1
Asks patient about tetanus	1
Asks patient about anticoagulation	1
Explains procedure	2
Selects steristrips	1
Uses clean technique	1
Carries out thorough saline lavage	1
Follows correct technique:	
• Closely opposes wound edges	1
• Applies steristrips to wound	1
• Achieves adequate closure	1
• Applies non-adherent dressing	1
Warns to keep dry	1
Warns about signs of infection	1
Asks about relevant medical history, e.g. peripheral vascular disease, diabetes	1
Advises when to return if worried, and advises about the risks of a non-healing wound requiring skin graft	1
Invites questions	1
Global score from examiner	5
Global score from actor	5
Total	**29**

Question 97 Seizure 4

Instructions for candidate

You are called to see an elderly lady who has just had an injection of local anaesthetic into her hand during the process of having manipulation of her forearm fracture using regional anaesthesia (Bier's block). The nurse tells you that she has noticed that the cuff on the equipment is deflated, and the patient reported feeling very unwell and then started to have a seizure.

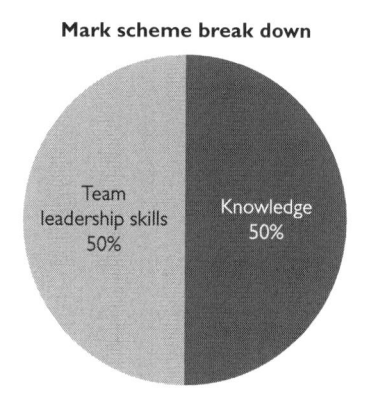

Mark scheme break down

- Team leadership skills 50%
- Knowledge 50%

Instructions for actor

You are an experienced ED nurse, but you have not seen this happen before. You noticed that the cuff on the Bier's machine was not inflated, shortly before your patient had a seizure. You follow the instructions of the candidate. Please do not prompt.

Instructions for examiner

You may provide the candidate with the following information if requested:

Tonic-clonic movements visible
A—airway clear
B—SaO_2 = 80% on air, 93% on high-flow O_2
C—HR = 160, BP = 80/40, CRT = 4 seconds
D—GCS 3, blood glucose = 10
Seizure continues despite treatment for 5 minutes

Equipment required

Standard adult resuscitation equipment (see introductory section)
Bier's block machine

Curriculum mapping

Sections of the CEM (2010) curriculum relevant to this question include the following.

Common competencies

CC1 History taking
CC2 Clinical examination
CC3 Therapeutics and safe prescribing
CC4 Time management and decision-making

CC5 Decision-making and clinical reasoning
CC6 Patient as the central focus of care
CC7 Prioritization of patient safety in clinical practice
CC8 Team work and patient safety
CC9 Principles of safety and quality improvement
CC14 Complaints and medical error
CC15 Communication with colleagues and cooperation

ACCS Acute presentations CT1&2

CAP15 Fits/seizure
CAP23 Pain management
CAP27 Poisoning
CAP33 Traumatic limb and joint injuries

Guidelines available

http://www.collemergencymed.ac.uk/shop-floor/clinicalguidelines/, then follow **Intravenous Regional Anaesthesia for Distal Forearm Fractures (Bier's Block)**

Mark scheme

Introduces self	1
Takes focused history of events from nurse	2
Gives oxygen	1
Follows A B C D E approach	2
Inserts NP airway	1
Makes diagnosis of local anaesthetic toxicity	1
Calls for senior ED help	1
Calls for anaesthetic assistance	1
Reinflates cuff	1
Checks blood glucose	1
Gives IV bolus of fluid (500 ml or 1000 ml of normal saline)	1
Requests/gives intralipid	3
Considers RSI	1
Displays team leadership skills	2
Global score from examiner	5
Global score from actor	5
Total	**29**

Question 98 Septic screen

Instructions for candidate
You are working in a paediatric ED. You have been seeing a 4-week-old baby who has a fever, of unknown source, who is reasonably well otherwise. You need to do a septic screen on the baby. Please discuss this with the parents. You are not expected to do any practical procedures in this station.

Mark scheme break down

- Knowledge 50%
- Communication 50%

Instructions for actor
You are the mother of a 4-week-old baby, Millie, who has been completely well until today. She was born 3 days earlier than expected, in a normal delivery. This morning when you put her down for a sleep, you noticed she felt hot and sweaty and her face was very red. You took her to your GP an hour later who took a temperature and found that it was 38.6°C. The GP then sent you to the paediatric ED.

Millie has been feeding well today, but she has been a little bit sleepier. She has been otherwise completely normal. She has not had any immunizations yet. She is your only child. There are no illnesses in the family. You expected to come to hospital for 'a check up' and be sent home again. You don't understand why all these tests are required. You are especially worried about Millie having an LP. When it is all explained to you, you consent to whatever is advised.

Instructions for examiner
Observation only.

Equipment required
None

Curriculum mapping
Sections of the CEM (2010) curriculum relevant to this question include the following.

Common competencies
CC5 Decision-making and clinical reasoning
CC6 Patient as the central focus of care
CC10 Infection control
CC12 Relationship with patients and communication
CC13 Breaking bad news
CC18 Valid consent

Paediatric acute presentations (PAPs)

PAP9 Fever in all age groups
PAP13 Neonatal presentations

Mark scheme

Introduces self, checks mother's identity	1
Uses open question to start	1
Asks what mother understands so far/recaps situation	1
Provides adequate explanation of septic screen:	1
• Unknown source of infection	1
• Important to treat correctly	1
• Neonatal infection risks	1
Explains different components:	
• Bloods	1
• LP	1
• Urine, by catheter or suprapubic catheter	1
• +/– CXR	1
Explains LP in detail:	
• Positioning	1
• Procedure	1
• After care	1
• Complications and risks	1
Gives advice about results and ongoing plan	2
Invites questions	1
Addresses concerns/answers questions	1
Global score from examiner	5
Global score from actor	5
Total	**28**

Question 99 Syncope

Instructions for candidate

This 16-year-old girl has collapsed at school and has been brought to hospital by ambulance. She is now conscious. She has been seen by a triage nurse, who has done a BP, HR, blood glucose, SaO_2, and ECG, which are all normal. Please take a history and explain to the patient what your management plan is.

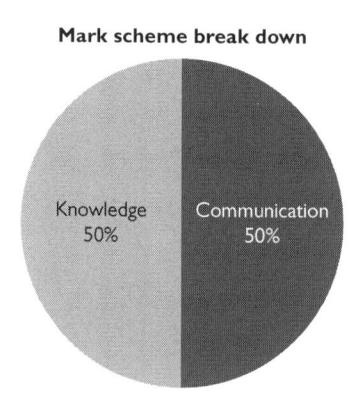

Mark scheme break down

- Knowledge 50%
- Communication 50%

Instructions for actor

You are a 16-year-old girl who has just fainted at school. You were standing in your biology lesson, watching the teacher dissect an animal heart. You felt hot and sweaty, and could feel your heart racing. You felt sick but didn't vomit. Your hearing and vision went 'funny' and then you fell forward onto another pupil, and slid down onto the floor and blacked out.

You can't remember how long you were unconscious for, but your friends said you were unresponsive for a few seconds and then you came round. They also say you looked very pale and sweaty. You didn't wet yourself, bite your tongue, or make any funny movements. You tried to sit up straight away, but you felt weak and dizzy again. You were given a glass of milk by the teacher. After about 15 minutes of lying down you felt back to normal. You are keen to go home.

You have had a tracing of your heart (ECG) which the nurse told you was ok. You didn't have any chest pain, breathing difficulties, or weakness in any part of your body. You have never had sexual intercourse, so you cannot be pregnant. You have never fainted before, but you always feel sick at the sight of blood. You did not have any breakfast today because you were running late. You have no medical problems and take no medication.

Instructions for examiner

Observation only.

Equipment required

Normal ECG

Curriculum mapping

Sections of the CEM (2010) curriculum relevant to this question include the following.

Self-Assessment for the MCEM Part C

Common competencies

CC1 History taking
CC4 Time management and decision-making
CC5 Decision-making and clinical reasoning
CC6 Patient as the central focus of care
CC11 Management of long-term conditions and promoting patient self-care
CC12 Relationship with patients and communication

ACCS Acute presentations CT1&2

CAP32 Syncope and presyncope

Guidelines available

http://www.collemergencymed.ac.uk/shop-floor/clinicalguidelines/, then follow **CEM Summary of NICE *Guideline* CG109**

Mark scheme

Introduces self	1
Establishes reason for attendance	2
Takes thorough history of presenting complaint:	
• Preceding symptoms	2
• During the collapse	2
• Recovery period	2
Asks about previous history of similar episodes	1
Excludes specific symptoms:	
• Cardiovascular	1
• Neurological	1
Establishes pregnancy unlikely	1
Asks about dietary history	1
Asks about alcohol history	1
Asks about drug use	1
Asks about medications	1
Obtains past medical history	1
Shows patient ECG and describes it as normal	1
Diagnoses simple vasovagal episode and explains this	2
Advises pregnancy test	1
Advises can be discharged after examination	1
Global score from examiner	5
Global score from actor	5
Total	**36**

Question 100 Foreign body removal

Instructions for candidate

This 2-year-old child has been brought to the ED because her parents have noticed that there seems to be a bead inside her left nostril. Please examine the child and then remove the foreign body, using the equipment available. You have a nurse to assist.

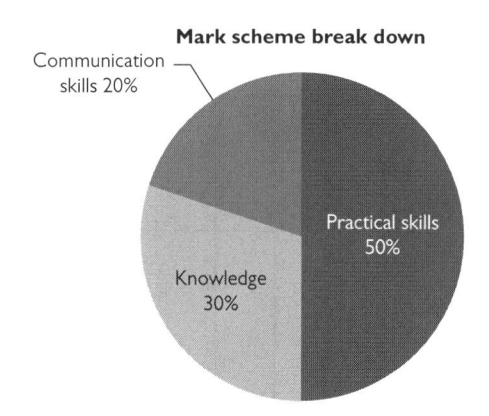

Mark scheme break down
- Communication skills 20%
- Knowledge 30%
- Practical skills 50%

Instructions for actors

You noticed today that your 2-year-old had something brightly coloured up her left nostril. She had been playing at a friend's house yesterday and there were some beads there, so you think it may be that. She seems to be absolutely fine. She has not had any episode of coughing or choking. She has never done this before. She is normally fit and well. You are willing to hold your child as instructed, to help get the bead out.

Instructions for examiner

At the end of the station, if the candidate is successful in removing the bead, ask the candidate what they would do if they were unable to extract the bead.

Equipment required

Infant manikin with foreign body in nostril
Nasal speculum
Light source
Forceps—selection of sizes and types
Hook
Suction and selection of suction catheters
Self-inflating BVM device

Curriculum mapping

Sections of the CEM (2010) curriculum relevant to this question include the following.

Common competencies

CC5 Decision-making and clinical reasoning
CC12 Relationship with patients and communication

CC15 Communication with colleagues and cooperation
CC18 Valid consent

Paediatric acute presentations (PAPs)

PAP8 ENT

Mark scheme

Introduces self	1
Washes hands	1
Examines child to confirm foreign body present	1
Instructs parents to try nose blowing with one nostril occluded	2
Instructs parents to try 'parent's kiss' technique and can do this with BVM	2
Explains to parents and child technique for removal using instruments	1
Explains position of child with arms temporarily restrained	1
Selects suitable equipment	1
Gets assistant from nursing staff where needed	1
Applies appropriate technique for removal of foreign body	1
If unable to remove foreign body, suggests ENT referral	1
Is reassuring and sympathetic throughout	1
Global score from examiner	5
Global score from actors	5
Total	**24**

Index

A

abdominal aortic aneurysm (AAA) 120, 153–4
abdominal examination
  chest pain 18
  in child 157–88
abdominal fluid 138, 139
abdominal pain 26, 27, 151–4
  central line 197
  drug abuse 151–2, 197–8
  femoral line 78
  haematemesis 213–14
  sickle cell disease 34
  ultrasound imaging 138–9
abscess, finger 28
accessory nerve 112
Achilles' tendon tear 191
acromioclavicular joint (ACJ) 50, 51
acuity, visual 91, 92, 112
acute angle closure glaucoma 92
adrenaline 15, 102, 162, 200
  anaphylaxis 169, 170
airway management 83–5, 168
  poisoning 182
  sepsis 187
  thunderclap headache 123–4
alcohol use
  chest pain 38, 39
  driving advice 211–12
  overdose 52–3
  sexual behaviour 11–12
  travel-induced disorder 27
alfentanil 123
anaemia 59
anaesthesia
  general 126
  local 24, 29
  rapid sequence induction of anaesthesia (RSI) 123, 176
  regional 133–5, 219
analgesia
  abdominal pain 151
  analgesic ladder 152
  ankle injury 116
  drug abuse 34, 35
  ear pain 73
  forearm fractures 32, 33
  headache 71
  knee joint aspiration 47
  lacerations, forearm 55
  local 47

shoulder examination 50, 51
wrist injury 37, 118
anaphylaxis 169–70
anatomy, ECG interpretation 188
aneurysm
  abdominal aortic 120, 153–4
  cardiovascular examination 18
  infra-renal aortic 194–6
angiogram 70
ankle injury 136–7
  fracture 115–16
anterior superior iliac spine 160
antibiotic requesting 171–2
antibiotic treatment 176, 187
anticoagulation 214, 218
antidepressant overdose 181–3
antimalarials 26, 27
antiplatelet agents 214
anti-sickness medication 71
aortic aneurysm 194–6
aortic valve, auscultation 17
apex, auscultation 17
appetite loss 26
arm weakness 81
arrhythmias 189
arterial line 149–50
aseptic technique
  catheterization 20
  chest aspiration 24
  intraosseus access 216
  paronychia 29
aspiration
  chest 23–5
  knee joint 46–7
asthma 65–6, 136, 147–8
asystole 199–200
atrial fibrillation 113
auroscopy 48–9
auscultation 15, 17, 18, 59
axis 189

B

back blows, choking 102
backslab placement 116
bad news, breaking
  cerebral metastases 192–3
  intracranial bleed in elderly patient 30–1
  road accident 63–4
  see also communication skills
bag valve mask (BVM) 83
bandaging 33, 116, 122

Index

barrier protection, failure to use 11–12, 109–10
basic life support 140–1, 163
benzodiazepine 176
beta human chorionic gonadotrophin (BHCG) 120
bicarbonate 15
Bier's block 133, 219
bilateral chest drains 63
blame, accepting 37
bleeding
    haematemesis 213–14
    intracranial 30–1
    risk factors 214
    upper gastrointestinal 103–4
    vaginal 177–8
blood cultures 187
blood gas analysis 207–8
blood pressure
    chest aspiration 24
    chest pain 69
    pre-eclampsia 88
blood transfusion
    Jehovah's Witness 103–4
    road accident 63
blood-borne viruses 12, 205, 206
body language 22, 31, 172
bougie 84
breathing assessment 168
breathing difficulties *see* shortness of breath (SOB)
bupivacaine 47
burns 167–8
    in child 60–2

C

caesarean section, perimortem 94
CAGE screening test 12
calf swelling 190, 191
cancer 107–8, 192–3
cannula use 47, 206
capacity 103–4
capnography 85
cardiac arrest
    asystole 200
    blood gas analysis 207–8
    choking 102
    neonatal resuscitation 163
    in pregnancy 93, 94
    road accident 63
cardiac enzymes 38, 70
cardiac monitoring 182
cardiac risk factors 70
cardiopulmonary resuscitation (CPR) *see* CPR (cardiopulmonary resuscitation)
cardiovascular examination 16–18
catheterization 19–20
    central line 198

femoral line 79
    sepsis 187
cauda equina 120
cell count 47, 160
central cord syndrome 82
central line 197–8
cerebral metastases 192–3
cerebrospinal fluid (CSF) 160
cervical spine
    collar, removal 128–9
    computerized tomography (CT) scan 42
    examination 51
chemotherapy 108
chest aspiration 23–5
chest compressions 15, 141
chest drain 99, 142–4
chest expansion, symmetrical 59
chest pain 16, 38–9, 69–70
chest percussion 59
chest thrusts, choking 102
chest X-ray (CXR) 23, 25, 85
    chest drain 144
    performed in error 36
    sepsis 187
child protection 60–2
chlorphenamine 170
choking 101–2
cholesterol, high 113
closed circuit television (CCTV) cameras 44
cluster headaches 72
cocaine 38, 39
Colles fracture, displaced 133–5
communication skills
    child protection issues 62
    empathy 178
    and Jehovah's Witness 104
    non-judgemental attitude 152, 166
    non-verbal 22, 31, 172
    open/closed questions 39, 61, 154
    orientation questions 185
    plain language 31, 64
    silence, appropriate use 31, 64
    specific disorder or procedure
        asthma management 66, 148
        chest aspiration 25
        elbow injury 21–2
        knee joint aspiration 47
        X-ray of wrong type performed in error 37
    team leadership 85, 168, 170, 183, 200, 220
    understanding of procedure, checking 47, 55, 81, 97, 114, 118
    see also bad news, breaking; reassurance
Community Psychiatric Nurse (CPN) 44
complaint, formal 36–7
computerized tomography (CT) scan

bleeding and swelling on brain 145
cerebral metastases 192, 193
cervical spine 42
consciousness, reduced level 100
headache, severe 72
intracranial bleed 30, 31
subarachnoid haemorrhage 159
consciousness, reduced level 98, 100
burns 167, 168
see also unconsciousness
contraception, emergency 11–12
cord compression 82
corneal reflex 112
cough 102
CPR (cardiopulmonary resuscitation)
asystole 200
choking 102
hypothermia 162
neonatal resuscitation 164
shortness of breath, in pregnancy 95
cranial nerves 111–12
cruciate ligaments 68
Cusco speculum 174
cyanosis 59

D

deep vein thrombosis (DVT) 190–1
dehydration 75, 203–4
delay in presentation 61
delayed cardiac enzymes 70
developmental milestones 74
dexamethasone 108
dextrose 15
dialysis, renal 56
diarrhoea 26, 27, 75–7, 175
dehydration 203–4
diazepam, rectal 175
differential diagnosis, shortness of breath 57
digital nerves 118
direct current (DC) shock 182
discharge advice 25, 65
distal radial fracture 117
undisplaced 32–3
distal tibia/fibula, fracture 115
driving advice 132, 211–12
drug abuse
abdominal pain 151–2, 197–8
chest pain 38–9
sickle cell disease 34–5
Drug and Alcohol Support Team 211
dyspnoea see shortness of breath (SOB)
dysuria 109–10

E

ear, nose, and throat (ENT) 171
ear pain 73–4

eclamptic seizure 86–8
effusion, atraumatic 46–7
elbow
injury 121–2
pulled 21–2
electrocardiogram (ECG) 40–1
chest aspiration 24
chest pain 38
interpretation 188–9
syncope 223
emergency contraception 11–12
end tidal carbon dioxide ($ETCO_2$) 84
end-of-life decisions 30, 31
endoscopic retrograde cholangiopancreatography (ERCP) 186
endoscopy 214
endotracheal tube (ETT) 84
entonox 116, 126
ephedrine 124
epilepsy 130–2, 134, 165–6
epilim 165
EpiPen® 170
equipment
adult 9
arterial line 149–50
auroscope/otoscope 48–9
endotracheal tube 84
laryngoscope 84
manometer 160
nebulizer 65
ophthalmoscope 96–7
paediatric 9–10
resuscitation 9–10
errors, explaining 36–7
erythropoietin (EPO) 104
examination
abdomen 157–88
ankle injury 137
cardiovascular 16–18
eye 91–2
hand 17, 59, 155–6
knee 67–8
limp, in child 106
lower limb 113
mental state 184–5
neurological 72
neurovascular 68
pelvic 173–4
respiratory system 58–9
shoulder 50–1
upper limb 82, 113
extradural haemorrhage 42
eye
examination 91–2, 112
yellow 209

Index

F

facial examination 17, 112
facial wound 201–2
family members, requests for 31
FAST (focused assessment with sonography for trauma) scan 120, 138, 194
febrile convulsion 179–80
femoral line 78–80
femoral pulses, cardiovascular examination 18
fentanyl 123
fertility treatment 177
fever 26, 73
fluid, in abdomen 139
fluid balance, checking 57
fluid bolus 99, 168, 170, 182, 187, 220
focused assessment with sonography for trauma (FAST) scan 120, 138, 194
forearm fracture 32–3
foreign body 225–6
fovea, retina 97
fractures
    ankle 115–16
    Colles fracture, displaced 133–5
    forearm 32–3
    missed 82
    neck of femur (NOF) 205–6
    olecranon, undisplaced 121–2
functional assessment, hand pain 156
fundoscopy 92, 97

G

gag reflex 112
gait assessment 113
gallstones 186
gastrointestinal complaints
    abdominal pain 151–4
    diarrhoea and vomiting 75–7
    gastroenteritis 151, 204
general anaesthesia (GA) 126
genito-urinary medicine (GUM) 12
Glasgow Coma Scale (GCS) 42, 43
Global Scoring Matrix 7, 8
glyceryl trinitrate (GTN) spray 69, 70
gout 47
guide wire
    central line 198
    femoral line 79
gynaecology, emergency 11–12
    obstetric 86–8

H

haematemesis 213–14
haematological disorders
    anaemia 59
    haematemesis 213–14
    sickle cell disease 34–5
    see also bleeding
haemothorax 142–4
hand examination 17, 59, 155–6
hand washing 20
handover 119–20
headache 27, 71–2
    cerebral mass 107–8
    in pregnancy 86
    thunderclap 123–4
hearing, testing 112
heart rate (HR), in newborn 13, 15
hepatitis 12, 210
hepatomegaly 18
heroin 209
hip rotation, in child 105–6
history, checking
    abdominal pain 152
    ankle injury 137
    chest pain 39, 70
    child protection issues 61
    diarrhoea and vomiting 75
    drug abuse 35
    ear pain 74
    epilepsy 166
    headache 72
    jaundice 210
    limp, in child 106
    psychiatry 44
    seizure 87, 131
    shortness of breath 56, 57
    suicide risk assessment 53, 90
    travel-induced disorder 27
HIV risk 12, 205
hydrocortisone 170
hypertension 69, 71, 113, 153
hypertonic saline 124
hypoglycaemia 176
hypo/hyperkalaemia 95
hypotension 95
hypothenar eminence 156
hypothermia 95, 161–2
hypovolaemia 168
hypoxia 95

I

ibuprofen, overdose 52
immobilization of patient 81, 99, 133, 168
immunization history 26, 27, 74, 75, 110
impingement tests 51
in vitro fertilization (IVF) 177
infants, resuscitation 163–4
infection, warnings about 55
inflation breaths 15
infra-renal aortic aneurysm 194–6

inhaler technique 65–6, 147–8
injuries
    ankle 136–7
    elbow 121–2
    neck 81–2, 127–9
    needlestick 205–6
    wrist 32, 117–18
instability tests 51
Intensive Therapy Unit (ITU) 31
intercostal chest drain 142–4
intercostal space
    chest aspiration 24
    chest pain 41
internal jugular vein 198
intracranial bleed 30–1
intralipid 220
intra-muscular (IM) naloxone 83
intraosseus access 215–16
intravenous (IV) drug use 12, 34, 78–80
intravenous (IV) fluids 34, 78, 170
introducers 198
intubation 15, 43, 63, 95, 99, 102, 162
    airway skills 83, 84
    anaphylaxis 168, 169
inversion injury 136–7

J
jaundice 209–10
Jehovah's Witness 103–4
jugular venous pressure (JVP) 17

K
ketamine 125
kidney, transplant 56
knee examination 67–8
knee joint aspiration 46–7

L
lacerations, forearm 54–5
lactate 181
language skills 31, 64
laryngeal mask airway (LMA) 83, 84
laryngoscope 84
last menstrual period 11–12
lateral collateral ligament stress test 68
left-sided weakness 113–14
lignocaine 24, 29, 47, 143
limp, in child 105–6
liver disorders 12, 209–10
local anaesthesia
    chest aspiration 24
    chest drain 143
    femoral line 79
    intraossseus access 216
    knee joint aspiration 47
    lumbar puncture 160
    paronychia treatment 29
    suturing 55
    toxicity 220
log roll 128
lumbar puncture 72, 159–60, 222
lymph nodes, enlarged 59

M
macula, retina 97
magnetic resonance imaging (MRI) 82
malaria 26, 27
mannitol 124
manometer 160
manubrio-sternal junction 143
McMurray's test 68
medial collateral ligament stress test 68
medial nerve distribution 117, 118
median nerve motor 156
medication, refusal to take 165, 166
Membership of the College of Emergency Medicine
    (MCEM) examination
    approach 1–2
    format 2–5
menstrual period 11–12
mental health disorders 44–5
mental state examination 184–5
metacarpal-phalangeal joint (MCPJ) 33, 116
methadone 34, 35, 209
methamoglobinaemia 134
metoraminol 124
microscopy, culture and sensitivity (MCS) 160
migraine 72
mini mental state examination 184–5
miscarriage 177–8
mitral valve, auscultation 17
mood disorders 44–5
morning after pill (MAP) 11–12
morphine 34, 35, 151, 152
mosquito bites 26
movement, joint 51, 68
muscle relaxant 84

N
naloxone 83
nasophyngeal (NP) airway 84
National Institute for Health and Care Excellence
    (NICE) 172
nebulizer 65
neck
    injury 81–2, 127–9
    inspection/palpation 59
neck of femur (NOF), fracture 205–6
needlestick injury 205–6
    avoidance while suturing 55

Index

neonatal resuscitation 13–15, 163–4
neurological examination 72
neurosurgical referral 42–3
neurovascular examination 68
neurovascular supply, distal 33
newborn, resuscitation 13–15
non-accidental injury (NAI) 106
non-invasive blood pressure (NIBP) 124
non-judgemental attitude 152, 166
non-steroidal anti-inflammatory drugs (NSAIDs) 47
non-verbal communication skills 22, 31, 172
nose blowing 226
numbness, in arms 81

O

Objective Structural Clinical Examination (OSCE)
    do's and don'ts 6–7
    format 2–6
obstetric emergency 86–8
oedema
    cardiovascular examination 18
    cerebral mass 107–8
    deep vein thrombosis 191
    shortness of breath 57
olecranon fracture, undisplaced 121–2
olfactory symptoms 112
ophthalmoscopy 96–7
    eye examination 96–7
opiates 84
oral endotracheal tube (OETT) 124
oral fluid regime 203, 204
organ donation 64, 145–6
organ donation register 63, 145
organisation skills 51, 59, 137, 174, 191
oropharyngeal (OP) airway 84
oropharynx 124
osteoporosis 30
otoscope 48–9
Ottawa ankle rules 137
overdose 52–3, 120
    poisoning 181–3
    risk assessment 89–90
oxygen, administering 99, 162, 168, 176, 220

P

P waves 189
Paddington screening test 12
paediatric acute presentations (PAPs)
    asthma 147
    facial wound 201
    febrile convulsion 180
    limp 106
    and septic screen 222
    trauma 99
Paediatric Intensive Care Unit (PICU) 102

paediatric major presentations (PMPs)
    febrile convulsion 180
    intraosseous access 215
    resuscitation 164
    trauma 99
paediatric medicine
    abdominal examination 157–88
    child protection 60–2
    choking 101–2
    diarrhoea and vomiting 75–7
    ear pain 73–4
    equipment 9–10
    falls 125–6
    febrile convulsion 179–80
    inhaler technique 147–8
    limp, in child 105–6
    resuscitation 13–15, 163–4
    seizure 175–6
    septic screen 221–2
    trauma 98–100
pain
    abdominal 26, 27, 151–4
    chest 38–9, 69–70
    ear 73–4
    eyes 91
    hand 155–6
    headache 71–2
    management see analgesia
    nature 72
pallor 38
palpation
    abdomen 158
    hand 156
    knee 68
    pulse 17
    shoulder 51
    symmetrical chest expansion 59
palpitations 38, 40
pancreatitis 78, 197
paracetamol
    blood testing for 52
    overdose 89–90
paranoia 44, 45
'parent's kiss' technique 226
Parkland fluid formula 168
paronychia 28–9
partial pressure of carbon dioxide (pCO_2) 181
partial pressure of oxygen (pO_2) 181
pastoral support 64
patella apprehension test 68
peak flow monitor 65
pelvic examination 173–4
permissive hypotension 194, 196
phenytoin 176
pilocarpine drops, eyes 92

plaster cast 32, 33, 116
plaster of Paris 121
pneumothorax 23, 24, 95
poisoning 181–3
polycystic renal disease 56
PR interval 189
precordium, inspecting 17
prednisolone, oral 147
pre-eclampsia 86–8
pregnancy
   pre-eclampsia 86–8
   shortness of breath 93–5
   see also neonatal resuscitation
pregnancy testing 12
prevention inhalers 66
prodromal symptoms (warning signs) 131
prognosis, poor 30, 31
propofol 84, 124
prostate, enlargement 19
proteinuria 87
psychiatry 44–5
'pulled elbow' 21–2
pulmonary embolism (PE) 120
pulmonary oedema 57
pulmonary valve, auscultation 17
pulse, examination 17, 18, 59
pupil reactions, assessment 92, 112
pus, expressing 29

Q
QRS waves/length 189
QT interval 189
quality of life 31
questioning skills 39

R
radial nerve distribution 118
radial nerve motor 156
radiotherapy 108
rapid sequence induction of anaesthesia (RSI) 123, 176
Raynaud's phenomenon 134
reassurance 20, 22, 28
regional anaesthesia 133–5, 219
rehydration salt solution 77
renal dialysis 56
rescue breaths 141
respiratory rate (RR) 59
respiratory system, examination 58–9
responsibility, taking 37
resuscitation
   cardiopulmonary 95
   ceasing 63
   equipment 9–10
   Intensive Therapy Unit (ITU) 31
   neonatal 13–15, 163–4

retained products, in miscarriage 178
retina, imaging 97
rewarming 162
Rhinnes hearing test 112
ring block, paronychia 29
ring-enhancing lesions 192
risk assessment, overdose 89–90
road accidents 63–4, 127–9
Rockall score 214

S
SADPERSONS scale, suicide risk assessment 53, 90
salbutamol 65, 66, 136, 147, 170
salicylate, blood testing for 52
saline lavage 55, 202, 218
SBAR (situation, background, assessment, recommendation) 95
scalp bruising 42
scalpel use 29, 79, 143
scar formation 202
sedation 125–6
seizure
   alcohol withdrawal 211
   cerebral mass 107
   epilepsy 130–2, 165–6
   febrile convulsion 179–80
   frequency 166
   in pregnancy 86
   regional anaesthesia 219–20
   in young child 175–6
sepsis 186–7
   septic screen 221–2
sexual lifestyle 12, 109–10
sexually transmitted diseases 11–12, 109–10
shivering 26
shocks 162
shortness of breath (SOB) 25, 56–7
   asthma 65–6, 147–8
   in pregnancy 93–5
shoulder examination 50–1
sickle cell disease 34–5, 134
sight, problems with 72, 91–2
silence, appropriate use 31, 64
slings 33, 51, 122
slurred speech 72
smoking history 39, 109, 209
sodium bicarbonate 182, 183
spacers 147
sport-related issues 67, 68
sternocleidomastoid nerve 112
stroke 71
subarachnoid haemorrhage 72, 159
suicide attempts 52–3, 89–90
suturing 54–5
   fall, in child 125, 126
   femoral line 79

Index

suxamethonium 84, 124
syncope 223–4

T

T waves 189
tachycardia 98, 167
tamponade 95
team leadership skills 85, 168, 170, 183, 200, 220
tension headache 72
tension pneumothorax 95
tetanus vaccination 55, 168
thenar eminence 156
thiopentone 124
thromboembolic fracture 95
thunderclap headache 123–4
tongue movement 112
tonic clonic movements 175
transducer, arterial line 150
transplant, kidney 56
trauma, paediatric 98–100
travel-induced disorder 26–7, 110
tricuspid valve, auscultation 17
trochar 216
troponin 69, 70
Tubinette™ gauze layers 33, 116

U

ulnar nerve distribution 118
ulnar nerve motor 156
ultrasound 138–9
    arterial line 150
umbilical venous access 15
unconsciousness
    assault 42
    intracranial bleed 30–1
    road accident 63
    see also consciousness, reduced level
upper gastrointestinal (GI) bleed 103–4
upper GI endoscopy 214
upper limb weakness 81, 82, 113, 114
upper respiratory tract infection 171–2, 179–80
urate crystals 47
urethritis, non-specific 110

urinary problems
    dysuria 109–10
    urine retention 19–20
urine sample 187
urology, catheterization 19–20

V

vaginal bleeding 177–8
valve auscultation 17
vasopressor 124
vasospasm 38
vasovagal episode, simple 224
Velband 122
venous blood gas (VBG) 120
ventilation 15
    bag valve mask 83
vestibulocochlear nerve 112
visual disturbance 72, 91–2
volumatic, in asthma 65, 66, 147, 148
vomiting 26, 72, 75–7, 175, 197
    of blood 213–14
    dehydration 203–4

W

Webers hearing test 112
Well's criteria 190
wheezing, in asthma 65
whiplash 129
white blood cells (WBCs), cell count 47, 160
wound closure 217–18
wrist injury 32, 117–18

X

xanthochromia 160
X-rays
    central cord syndrome 82
    chest X-ray 23, 25
    elbow injury 21
    forearm fracture 32, 33
    incorrect type performed in error 36–7
    lacerations, forearm 54

Y

yellow skin 209